DID YOU KNOW . . .

- 90 percent of women are more interested in sex than men?
- Men can teach themselves to have multiple orgasms?
- Women prefer sexy buttocks and a slim stomach to a large penis?
- 10–20 percent of women can climax by breast stimulation alone?
- Unmarried women usually fantasize about their boyfriends, while married women often fantasize about strangers?
- An oversized penis is worse for sex than an undersized one?
- A man should *never* promise a woman that he's going to make her come?
- Men can train themselves to keep going . . . for as long as she wants?

Don't let ignorance leave you out in the cold.
Become the hot lover you were meant to be with . . .

SATISFACTION GUARANTEED

SATISFACTION GUARANTEED

WHAT WOMEN
REALLY WANT IN BED

RACHEL SWIFT

WARNER BOOKS

A Time Warner Company

If you purchase this book without a cover you should be aware that this book may have been stolen property and reported as "unsold and destroyed" to the publisher. In such case neither the author nor the publisher has received any payment for this "stripped book."

PUBLISHER'S NOTE: All statistics refer to the United Kingdom.

The author and publishers wish to thank the following, who have kindly given permission for the use of copyright materials:
Edvard Dermit for the drawing by Jean Cocteau on page 102. From *The Passionate Penis*, published by Peter Owen Ltd.
Zygmunt Frankel for his poem "With All The," which was first published in *Slightly Nasty Poems*. It also appears in Fiona Pitt-Kethley's *The Literary Companion to Sex*.
Charles Thomson for the opening lines of his "Penis Poem," which was first published in Fiona Pitt-Kethley's *The Literary Companion to Sex*.
Every effort has been made to trace all copyright holders, but if any have been inadvertently overlooked, the author and publishers will be pleased to make the necessary arrangement at the first opportunity.

Warner Books Edition
Copyright © 1996 by Rachel Swift
All rights reserved.

This Warner Books edition is published by arrangement with Pan Books, an imprint of Macmillan Publishers, Ltd., London.

Warner Books, Inc., 1271 Avenue of the Americas, New York, NY 10020

Visit our Web site at www.twbookmark.com

 A Time Warner Company

Printed in the United States of America

First Warner Books Printing: January 2000

10 9 8 7 6 5 4 3 2 1

Library of Congress Cataloging-in-Publication Data

Swift, Rachel.
    Satisfaction guaranteed : what women really want in bed / Rachel Swift.
      p. cm.
    ISBN 0-446-67591-1
    1. Sex instruction for men.   2. Sex.   3. Sexual excitement.
  I. Title.   II. Title: What women really want in bed.
HQ36.S94   2000
306.7—dc21   99-36567
                                                    CIP

Book design by Nancy Singer

This book is dedicated to all the many
women and men
who wrote to me with their stories, tips, and opinions
after reading *How to Have an Orgasm . . . As Often As You
Want.*
(Names have been changed to protect identities.)

Acknowledgments

This book could not have been published without the support of people from all over the United States. In particular, my enthusiastic agent, Alison J. Picard; my editors and proofreaders at Warner Books, whose professionalism and efficiency have been a joy; and Lorrie Bunn and friends, for their helpful copyediting.

Contents

By Popular Demand . . .

*S*atisfaction *Guaranteed* reveals what women *really* want during sex. Backed up by the tips, stories, and confessions of hundreds of women from around the world, it gives explicit, practical, and sometimes shocking advice about how to be a satisfying lover.

Satisfaction Guaranteed covers every topic, from what type of man (and penis) women find most attractive, to how to perform perfect oral sex. There is a chapter describing how a man can stop himself ejaculating too soon and another on how men can teach themselves to have multiple orgasms. There are sections on women's secret fantasies, the best sexual positions for satisfying a woman, why and how women fake orgasms, what they think about anal sex, and, finally, how the really good lover should behave in the gentle, exhausted moments after sex is over.

Three years ago, I wrote *How to Have an Orgasm . . . As Often As You Want*. In addition to my 6-step Orgasm Plan I revealed that far from having an ideal time in bed, 70 percent of women have great difficulty getting satisfied. To my delight, the book struck a chord around the world. It was translated into seventeen languages, in seven different alphabets, and sold in umpteen different countries.

Within a week of publication I was receiving astonishingly frank letters from women of all ages and backgrounds revealing their secret needs and desires, and answering in great detail the questionnaire included in the book. Each letter has been a pleasure to read, from the Rollerblading redhead who loves sex and writes, "I'm always reading to learn, experiment, and entertain myself. My poor partner gets attacked that day 'cause I'm all worked up and need a release," to the ex-nun who recently left her order: she bought a newspaper that advertised a "Millionaire's Game," saw an article about *How to Have an Orgasm,* and thought she ought to learn about orgasm too.

One theme cropped up again and again. In *How to Have an Orgasm* I had included a chapter for men. But these women wrote: "One chapter! You should write a whole book for men!" Men wrote to me saying the same thing. Booksellers revealed that men were buying the book almost as much as women, usually sneaked across to the cashier's desk under a pile of more manly titles like *Know Your All-Terrain Vehicle* and *The Army Ranger Wilderness Survival Guide.* In the words of one frustrated correspondent, female sexuality is a "downright mystery."

This book was written, therefore, by popular demand. It is not just my book. It is a message from women to men the world over.

When quoting readers, I have changed their real names, and I have ensured that other distinguishing details have been changed.

Why Are There So Many Bad Lovers?

"What proportion of men are really good in bed?" I ask this question whenever I am with a group of women. Alas, the results are not encouraging: I've never had a figure higher than 30 percent.

There are, however, good reasons for this. The first and most pernicious is the idea that good lovemaking is instinctive, like eating. This is rubbish. *Sex* may be a basic instinct, but making love is an art. Both sexes have to learn it, and men more so than women, because women are more sexually complicated and more various.

Young men tend to have their early sexual experiences with girls of their own age or younger. Girls, in other words, who are not sure themselves what pleases them, or are not assertive enough to speak up about it. Even experienced women cannot be relied upon to educate their lovers. Ninety years after feminism became a major force, women today remain annoyingly unassertive in the bedroom: when Harry rubs at Susie's tenderest parts as vigorously as a belt sander, Susie merely grits her teeth, smiles bravely, and makes a mental note to avoid Harry next time.

Then there's the fact that men don't talk usefully to one another about sex; they don't share secrets. The most a man will do is sketch a sort of wiggly shape with both hands to indicate—you know—what the lovely Tootsie, um, er, looks like underneath that tracksuit she always wears. When someone asks him how Tootsie behaves in private, he only raises his eyes skyward and confides, "Whooaah." Women, on the other hand, are much more frank about the subject and learn all sorts of delicious secrets from one another. Because we find sex essentially rather funny, we've no desire to be coy or gruff about it in private. When I lived in London the women in the neighborhood would get together every two weeks to analyze their latest escapades, swap spicy sex tips, and even give demonstrations using cucumbers and bananas—how to apply the famous Butterfly Flick technique when performing oral sex, or how to roll on a condom while giving "maximum pleasure." Great stuff!

Much of the blame for bad sex must also go to sex manuals. Too many of them concentrate on making sex unusual, rather than ensuring that the quality is good. They push ahead to fancy work that is arousing for men, but not for women. Even the best books make serious mistakes. Most are written by men who cannot understand what sex is really like for women, or by therapists who are too soft-spoken and politically correct to speak the hard truth. Bernard Zilbergeld's otherwise good book *Men and Sex* advises that it is "highly improbable" a woman will climax if she hasn't done so after "ten to fifteen minutes." Rubbish! Kim Scapa's *Sex Tips for Boys* is cunning and inventive, but declares that premature ejaculation (which can be readily cured) should be treated merely as an embarrassment of riches—tell that to the girls! David Reuben's highly influential *Everything you always wanted to know about sex but were afraid to ask* insists that oral sex will make even the most sexually unresponsive woman fly into wild ecstasies. Nonsense! Oral sex is very pleasant, *if done well,* but it no more guarantees orgasm than a ten-inch penis does. Such books talk about what is *supposed* to happen, not what actually does. In sex manuals there is no embarrassment, no awkwardness, no distaste—the partners are always strong, supportive, and eloquent about their personal needs. Not so in real life. Helena writes:

> I have read a lot of books about sex in my time. I always feel they exist on a different plane to me, sort of in the way poetry exists on a different plane to everyday experience. I can recognize the things the writers are talking about but they've been smoothed down and turned into something remote.

Men today are more willing to please their partners than ever before: a good half of the letters I receive from women speak about "my sweet, caring man" and such endearments. And yet women still find it very difficult to communicate their sexual desires. "I feel too shy to sit my boyfriend down and tell him that there are several things he's doing wrong," writes

Shirley. Men must be told about *real* sex, with all its difficulties and subtleties—not about ideal, fictional sex.

How Important to a Woman Is Good Sex in a Relationship?

It varies enormously from person to person, but it is almost certainly more important than she lets on.

If you define sex in narrow terms, as stimulation of each other's loins, then sex is unimportant to a few, but important to many. Lack of sexual satisfaction, writes one reader, "makes me a BITCH." For another, good sex is so important that it's caused her to think twice about her current relationship:

> I have the most sensitive, caring, and understanding individual as a boyfriend and yet sex is presently only vaguely passable. My previous boyfriend, however, had little in common with me, preferred his books to anything I could offer and had very little intellectual respect for me. But sex with him was great; "gasping for more" springs to mind . . . I'm fearful that my lack of sexual fulfillment will turn me away from a man I love to someone who makes me cry but who can make me come in five seconds.

If you define sex in the way that women tend to see it—as the whole loving and emotional experience, from the first kiss, the touching, the closeness, right on through to the moment you lie side by side together afterward, then 99.9 percent of women want this very badly. Sylvia, who is in her early fifties, writes frankly of her own marriage:

> My husband has rather lost interest in sex no matter how I try and tempt him. I do get really annoyed some-

times when he doesn't respond. I have very often felt very desperate because, although he is a considerate lover, he is not very demonstrative and if he were more "physical" in the touching and kissing first, I'm sure it would be better. I have tried to explain that I need him to "love me" just by kissing me and touching me, but he is rather shy about anything to do with feelings at all. He has never been as keen on sex as I am, but he is getting worse, and I must admit some of the men at work look very tempting on some days!

A man doesn't have to be a big performer to make his partner happy. Even if penetrative sex is off the menu, there are plenty of other techniques that give great pleasure. There's not a woman on earth who doesn't regard kissing and embracing and lying in each other's arms as something highly pleasurable. Good sex is not the most important part of a relationship, but bad sex or no sex is often the cause of it breaking up.

It's not hard for a man to become a good lover. You don't have to acquire a sophisticated "technique." On the contrary, the self-styled Sexpert is a menace whom women are eager to avoid. He's the man who has "got women all figured out" (as he most likely puts it). He's had success (apparently) with scores of women, and now applies the same methods of lovemaking to all of them. He's not open to suggestion, and always thinks he knows best. Here is an example of one such abomination, described by his girlfriend:

I'm twenty-four and my boyfriend is thirty-three. Before we got together I had no problem with having orgasm. I tried to tell him what I like and what it would take for me to reach an orgasm, but every time I've tried he informs me that he's had more sexual experience than I have and he should know better than I what it takes to please a female. None of my other lovers had any problems with making me reach the orgasm platform.

All the good lover needs is, not technique, but a willingness to listen and to learn . . .

The Importance of Learning

Remember the film *Mutiny on the Bounty,* with Marlon Brando and Trevor Howard? There's a stunning scene in which the galleon arrives at a South Sea island, and the highly unprepossessing English sailors are greeted by swarms of luscious raven-haired island girls. To the sailors' disbelief, these sirens take a man each and inveigle them off into the undergrowth (Marlon Brando gets the chief's daughter). The scene, based on the true story of the *Bounty* mutiny in 1789, draws on the Polynesian traditions of free love and, more to the point here, female sexual satisfaction. I have always suspected that behind those bushes the sailors got their faces slapped. The island girls were accustomed to a society where young men are trained from an early age to bring women to orgasm, and would have got a rude shock when they discovered that there is no comparable Western tradition, especially not among sex-starved seamen.

It was reading about another Polynesian island called Mangaia that resulted in my writing *How to Have an Orgasm,* because it made me appreciate how important learning is for sexual satisfaction. On this delightfully civilized little island, sex is still treated like any other subject requiring practice and tutoring. A boy starts his sexual education at the age of thirteen or fourteen with an older, experienced woman. She teaches him the techniques of foreplay, cunnilingus, and how to treat the female body as an erogenous whole. The sole purpose of these arts is to arouse the woman sufficiently for intercourse, which then lasts a quarter to half an hour, during which she climaxes two or three times, and the male holds off until the end. Any man who does not give full satisfaction earns a bad reputation on the island and is avoided by the other women. Bliss!

Women in less advanced societies look to such places wistfully. Recently I asked a group of friends—all intelligent, forceful, and articulate—about their experiences with men. After hearing scores of stories about unsatisfactory sex, they all agreed: "If you want to be sure of a good lover, catch him when he's young, and train him up!" It wasn't that older men couldn't learn the art just as well, but that most of them were set in their ways and refused to budge.

Whatever your age, a willingness to discover what your particular partner needs is essential if you want to be satisfactory in bed. It's of no relevance whether or not you pleased your previous lover if your current one is unsatisfied. For every man, no matter what his experience, there is always more that he can learn. It is well worth his while: good lovers are rare, highly appreciated, and never forgotten.

2

Women Are More Interested in Sex Than Men

I know. I've asked several thousand women. The response has been overwhelming.

Less interested in sex? No. No. No. No. No. Get the picture?

Ever been to the women's locker rooms? "Worse" than listening to men! But women's upbringing and the world's attitude tells them to pretend they don't care.

Not my girlfriends! All we talk about is sex and how we can't get enough of it!

I think males start off more interested and women end up more interested.

Society has mentally made most women believe they are not physically made up to want sex as much as a man, so they don't. But in their natural, uncluttered state they want it just as much or more than any man.

His sexual response is quite apparent, whereas a woman will just feel the need in a less obvious manner.

Woman's sex drive is a hell of a lot higher. I've never found a man who can outlast me. But women let bad sex get to them more. It's insinuated that it's their fault, and they're accused of being frigid.

Regardless of age, nationality, or social circumstances, a full 90 percent of women were adamant: we are just as interested, if not considerably *more* interested, in sex than men. A recent English survey, Susan Quilliam's *Women on Sex,* found that over 68 percent of women want more sex than they currently get. The popular idea that men are the only lusty half of the species is obviously wrong, a legacy of the Victorian fiction that no decent woman enjoys sex. Ancient literature is full of references to women's raunchy sexuality. Historian Antonia Fraser tells us that "the potentially repetitious and thus demanding nature of the female orgasm was fully understood" in the seventeenth century.

And yet men's greatest complaint about women is that they don't want sex often enough! How can this be? Why are men complaining? Is it just a breakdown of communications? Now that Swift has brought the oddity to light, is there a worldwide orgy in the offing?

Thank God, no.

The key word is "interest." Women find sex *interesting*—they savor every detail of the whole experience, from start to finish: the long, slow erotic preliminaries, the mutual passion, the penetration, and especially the blissful afterglow. But the sex has to be good. Although most men are willing to have sex as often as women want it, not enough men know how to make love as women want it. For women *bad sex is much worse than no sex.*

The problem is that most men approach sex in terms of

quantity not quality. A long, intimate encounter is very nice if it happens, and if the fellow's got the patience for it, but the main thing is to satisfy the dull ache in the groin. As a consequence, more and more of the woman's energy goes into masturbation and imagining erotic situations, and less and less into putting up with the unsatisfactory fumblings she gets in the bedroom. "My friends and I talk about sex very often and on a very explicit level," writes one woman. "In our fantasies we are all very free and daring but when we talk about sex—the *action* of sex with another person, there is frequently a feeling of dissatisfaction—certainly from the longer established couples."

> Women are as interested in sex or more so than men. We want to make it a beautiful, intense, close, memorable experience as well as to be satisfied so we often put more planning or just more thought into what will happen and how. That is, if the woman has the courage or encouragement to be assertive.

> I believe when women are alone or in the right environment they are VERY interested in sex. They probably want it even more than men do but have to repress the feeling . . . If you feel sexy and feel valued by the man, you will want sex.

> The frills matter less to men—a woman is more likely to wait until the frills are also available.

> If my man would treat sex as a whole thing I'd be much keener to have it with him. He thinks of sex as five minutes and I think of it as touching and being close. I want to be fucked but properly, otherwise it's not worth it because I feel like only a tenth of me has taken part and the disappointment is hard to bear. Instead I go to sleep. What's in it for me, otherwise? I am thinking of taking a lover. I need proper, intimate sex desperately.

> I think women strive for sexual pleasure at least as
> much as men—but they may not appear to be as eager
> for intercourse because (if) it doesn't give them the sex-
> ual pleasure they strive for.

Many women have given up sex with men because it simply wasn't worth it. I regularly speak to them about their erotic
experiences, and they all agree: *at most two or three in every ten
men can be considered satisfying lovers.* The sex researcher
Shere Hite has warned that if this situation does not improve,
women will be forced to turn to other women to get their satisfaction.

The real frustration for women is that bad sex is so easily
avoided.

How?

Read on . . .

Women's Sexuality Is Completely Different from Men's

The old argument, invented in the radical 1960s, that we're sexually identical is dead. It has collapsed under the weight of
common sense and scientific evidence. In our hearts of hearts
we always knew that male-female sexual sameness is not, was
not, and never will be true. Ignore the differences and you will
have profound problems. Admit and understand them, and sex
for both women and men becomes infinitely more pleasurable.

For a woman, good sex begins long before she gets into
bed. Despite the sexual revolution, and the rapidly increasing
power and independence of women, we still place vastly more
emphasis than men on the emotional and sensual environment
in which lovemaking takes place. "Like all women," writes Han-
nah, a physical education teacher, "I don't really separate sex as
a thing from the rest of my relationship with a man, certainly

not in the same way a man does. The quality of sex depends on so much other stuff, such as how my man and me were getting on beforehand and whether I'm really on the same wavelength with him and how did I spend my day? Happy? Bored? Erotic? Sad? These are, for women, all a part of foreplay. That's the biggest way men and women are different, because men can separate the act from the circumstances in which the act takes place, which women cannot do." "With sex for a man," says Diane from Missouri, "there's a beginning, a middle, and an end. But with a woman it's more like a circle."

Again and again women remark that sex without some degree of emotional intimacy is unpleasant. A study of university students found that only 40 percent of men, *but a full 95 percent of women,* required emotional involvement as "always" or "most of the time" a prerequisite for having sex. Approximately twice as many women as men say they were in love with their first sexual partner. "Once you've found the right man," insists one forty-eight-year-old, "one that you can relate to on every level, spiritually, intellectually, emotionally, etc.—the sex is 100 percent better, 'cause sex is between the ears."

Women appear more emotional than men. However, the men with whom I have had deep and meaningful conversations about sex have revealed a lot of emotion; they just don't always show it. My current lover will sometimes sob in my arms after we've made love.

I think emotions affect men too, but maybe they block it out better.

Until women can fully appreciate the physical pleasure it is probably an emotional act for them. How could our conscience allow us to engage in this activity if there is no gain, be it emotional, monetary, abuse or physical pleasure?

We are all emotional about sex, women just vocalize it more.

I just want to say: sex is wonderful but with a mate you love, trust and respect it will be much better; but please make sure his feelings are the same! Once in a solid commitment, sex can and will be anything you want it to be . . . hot and steamy, slow and passionate . . . kinky, or anything you want.

It doesn't have to be love and promise of nuptials. Many women claim that the best sex is with casual friends and not someone they're head over heels in love with, because only then can they be truly relaxed with each other. What matters for women, whether during a one-night stand or a long-term relationship, is that the man is sympathetic and companionable, and does not treat sex simply as a route to ejaculation. A gorgeous specimen of masculinity can be a total turn-off if he doesn't also behave gorgeously, and the circumstances aren't arousing. It holds true in homosexual relationships as well. Lesbians place more value on expressing emotion and getting the context right than do gay men. As a result, lesbians are much less likely than gay men to have sex with strangers. This isn't soppiness, it's what it takes to make sex good for women. An unemotive cold screw holds little attraction, whether it leads to orgasm or not.

There's a story about Mick Jagger that illustrates the point well. A groupie fantasized about sleeping with him. She thought that would be the ultimate in sexiness. So she worked her way through all the lesser rock stars, imagining each time that it was Mick and not the lead singer from Dripping Tap, until she finally got herself in bed with the great sex bomb himself. The result? Total disappointment. She had to fantasize about making love to Mick Jagger even as she was actually making love to him. That was the only way she could get any pleasure out of it at all! The circumstances of reality didn't live up to the circumstances in her dreams, and so the sex was bad. Can you imagine a man going to bed with Pamela Anderson and complaining it was a terrible letdown because she hadn't seduced him in exactly the way he'd hoped? For men, sex with a woman they love may be much better and infinitely more profound than with a total stranger for whom they have no feeling; but it's still not bad with a stranger, even when standing up, pushed against the wall of a dark alley. Women, no matter how hard they try, can't bring themselves to feel the same. Dark-alley sex is dull and highly uncomfortable.

One of the most fundamental ways in which the sexes differ in their erotic responses is that women are slower to become aroused than men, both physically and psychologically. Josie is an eighteen-year-old hairdresser—tall, with shoulder-length dark hair and beautiful, expressive eyes—who was invited out by a carpenter called Gavin. They met at her place, flirted over a drink, and set off. A couple of hours later they were sitting in the movie theater when Gavin put his hand inside Josie's blouse and squeezed her breasts. She slapped his face and walked out of the theater. He followed, angry and perplexed, calling her a prude.

Josie is not a prude. As she explains, "I don't happen to find a theater very sexy. I liked Gavin a lot, and I was thinking about going to bed with him. But I can't switch on enormous sexual desire to order. It comes gradually, as the evening advances, the more time I spend with him. What he did was a turn-off, it was so coarse. I mean physically coarse. My reaction was nothing to do with morals."

Another example will bring back uncomfortable memories to thousands of women. Dickie and Shay met at a party given by an old school friend and immediately fell for each other. I was there too: they obviously couldn't take their eyes off each other. While the rest of us were distracted by "Rock around the Clock," they crept off upstairs to find a bedroom with a lock.

Once inside, however, things suddenly went wrong. Dickie indulged in a few moments' "warm-up" and then climbed on top of Shay and attempted to penetrate. She got angry and pushed him off, and they both sulked for the rest of the evening.

"It was agony," recollected Shay. "I just physically need something a little more. Just because Dickie feels my panties are slightly wet does not mean I'm altogether ready. I have other parts to my body too, I'm not just a cunt. But he couldn't appreciate this. He thought that I ought to get aroused as quickly as he did and took it as almost an insult when I didn't." Unless a woman actually asks you to get on top right away, you must assume she needs gentle, gradual sexual arousal. Fifty percent of painful intercourse could be avoided if more lovers understood this simple fact.

Women are not only slower to get aroused, but we are aroused by different things. We respond erotically to a wider variety of stimuli than men, incorporating a larger region of the body. A woman's skin is thinner and more sensitive than a man's, possibly because of her estrogen levels. The female's love of creams, potions, and massage oils is far more than concern with beauty. It feels gorgeous to have our skin stroked, especially when there are pleasant scents involved too. When women protest that their lovers don't touch them enough, it is the expression of an erotic thirst for which most men don't feel the need. Interestingly, our sensitivity during orgasm also appears, from subjective reports, to be different: "It goes beyond that of the genitals," write Dr. Robbins and Professor Jensen in the *Journal of Sex Research;* women "report floating, disconnected, letting-go sensations," which are comparatively rare in men.

Music is also extremely important to women's sexual responsiveness. In cultures and tribes the world over, both sexes *enjoy* music, but when used directly for erotic effect it is almost always the man who sings or plays to woo his beloved and get her in the mood. The main sexual stimulant for teenybopper girls, for example, is music and in particular the song lyrics. They both suggest an emotional context, which is highly erotic; sex itself, particularly the sort of adolescent sex such girls have to put up with, seems bland without this pleasant setting.

Most women prefer to make love in the dark or semidark—a fact that so impressed sex researcher Alfred Kinsey that he concluded women's nerve centers are fundamentally different from men's. Darkness of course hides beauty imperfections, but it also heightens our sense of touch, smell, and hearing. Visual stimulation, on the other hand, means much less to women than to men. College students around the world are regularly dragged off to take part in experiments to back up these claims, and the results are always the same. Men can get highly aroused just by what they see—sexy legs, big breasts, explicit pictures—but for women the mere sight of a man's body really isn't up to much. In teenagers' bedrooms, the boys will have erotic pinups of anonymous naked women. Male equivalents do nothing for girls, who idolize rock stars and actors, whom they get to know and read about as *individuals. Cosmopolitan* magazine experimented with nude male centerfolds but had to discontinue them because they bored and annoyed the readers. Porno mags for women have also discovered that the readers are more interested in sexy stories than pinup nudes. "I find myself unmoved by photographs of dangling penises in magazines," wrote one woman to the British magazine *Viva*. "For me, a stark, static posed young man with a 'say cheese' smile and an exposed cock is completely boring." Women find this one of the hardest things to make a man appreciate: no matter how much he pumps iron and does prick-extension exercises, his naked body strutting around the room is simply not arousing per se. The Chippendales are an obvious case in point: women rarely watch them to get turned on, but because they are a novelty, good for a giggle, and because male bodies are interesting.

Pressure to Have Sex Is Utterly Unsexy

Because men's and women's sexualities are so different, it's a great (though often made) mistake to assume that a women always wants to approach sex with as much forthrightness as a man does. This applies both to long-term relationships and to one-night stands.

> Because my husband is very casual about sex we have a wonderful sex life. It is a fun thing for us. Very mutual. We do it every night, but I never feel like I have to do it with him or else he'll get annoyed. I know lots of women whose sex life in their marriage is bad because the man just won't let up always trying to force sex to happen, instead of letting it be natural, mutual.

> My best husbands (I've had six!!) in bed have been the ones who don't make an issue out of sex. I've always been more relaxed and sexual with a man who isn't constantly trying to do sex with me, which is when I feel that I'm a thing instead of a person, a female.

Many a woman has been pleasantly anticipating a nice evening with a man she likes, hoping that it will eventually end between the sheets—only to be abruptly turned off when he becomes too eager, panting to get to the last stage with unseemly haste. Jackie, a thirty-four-year-old lawyer, went for an evening to the theater with Mark, an accountant whom she'd known for a few months. "We'd had some sexual contact earlier," explains Jackie,

> before we set off, kissing, which I enjoyed. Then he completely blew it. It was winter, dark out, and we were walking from the subway to the theater when we passed a doorway. He drew me aside for a moment,

which I thought was quite sexy, and we kissed there. It was warm and intimate. Then he started pressing his hard cock up against me, really hard. It was just too much for that situation. I no longer had any choice left about how the evening would end. Before then it had been sexy to think of possibilities. Now delicate, erotic possibilities were turned into a sexual certainty.

Such behavior makes sex feel like a clumsy affair. To go through with it would be as bad as going to bed with a man who made bad smells. Pressure reeks of quantity sex, not quality sex. Ninety-two percent of women quoted in the Hite Report on *Love, Passion and Emotional Violence* expressed outrage at the constant sexual pressure from men. Women writing to me confirm it. "If men only knew how many times I've been within an ace of going to bed with them," said Sue, "and then they've ruined it by making me feel under pressure."

Some women claim to be able to spot a great lover at ten paces. "If he's any good at sex at all," writes Tanya, thirty-seven, "you as a woman know it long before you begin fucking. A good man never makes you feel sex is what you've got to get as fast as possible. The whole experience is what matters. Like, there'll be an afternoon together and maybe you don't do anything more than touch hands. It's all a gradual buildup. Once we're fondling and that, I like it when he says how desperate he is for me. That's a turn-on. I like to think I make him like that. I don't want it from the start, though. That's boy's stuff. It turns me off. I want to be two people together, not two fucking machines." As another woman, quoted in Quilliam's survey of English women's sexual attitudes, puts it: "Yes, I do have sex on the first date. It happens quite often, depending on the man. If he thinks that I will sleep with him, then I don't. I like to surprise them. I like to be in control before sex." Sadie, a devastatingly attractive woman who runs a clothes shop, is also emphatic on this point:

I loathe going to parties and seeing married men ogle me. They demean themselves and it has little to do with me personally. Only really stupid women get off on that. I know one or two—women who have absolutely nothing else going for them. Of course I like being attractive to men, but I expect them to be a bit subtle about it. The man I notice is dignified, not drooling.

Boys and young men almost always fail to observe the no-pressure rule, and it is an enormous shock to a girl when she first discovers the untutored adolescent's attitude to sex. What she had imagined would be a sensual, enveloping, gradual experience turns out to be cold, pushy, and impersonal. Hence that peculiar adolescent foible, the pickup line: "Wanna see my marble collection?" "May I examine your private parts?" "I'm collecting pubic hairs. May I have one of yours?" Such comments hold absolutely no attraction for a woman at all. Yet the fellow who says them honestly expects that they will attack a woman's true animal nature and make her neck with him on the spot, because it is how he, in his fantasies, imagines being seduced. Sue Grafton's murder mystery *I Is for Innocent* contains a typical example of this confused idea. The narrator, private eye Kinsey Millhone, is visiting jail to get a written statement from a twenty-eight-year-old convict. He is "lean and long-waisted with hips so narrow they hardly held his pants up. He looked good in jail blue." She introduces herself and explains her purpose when he suddenly butts in:

> "You single?"
> I checked behind me. "Who, me?"
> He smiled the kind of smile you'd have to practice in the mirror, eyes boring into mine. "You heard me."
> "What's that got to do with it?"
> His voice softened to the coaxing tone reserved for

stray dogs and women. "Come on. Just tell me. I'm a nice guy."

I said, "I'm sure you're very nice, but it's none of your business."

This amused him. "How come you're afraid to answer? Are you attracted to me? Because I'm attracted to you."

"Well, you're very forthcoming and I appreciate that, Curtis. Uh, now, could you tell me about the time you spent with David Barney?"

He smiled faintly. "All business. I like that. You take yourself serious."

"That's right. And I hope you'll take me serious, too."

If a woman did this to a man, he'd be flattered. When a man does it to a woman, she feels sick.

By the same score, women find men who talk about sex all the time equally tedious (and sometimes threatening). Even if the man's as handsome as Adonis it's hard to be attracted to him under these conditions. In constantly bringing the subject up the sex bore makes it boring, from a woman's point of view. He might as well be talking about the new transmission in his Volvo. Far from creating an air of eroticism, we end up suspecting he can't get it up at all. Why would he be so obsessed with the subject otherwise? It was not for nothing that Gary Cooper based his legendary seduction technique on playing down the sexual side as much as possible. "If I ever saw him with a good-looking girl," remembered the film director Howard Hawks, "and he was kind of dragging his feet over the ground and being very shy and looking down, I'd say, 'Oh-oh, the snake's gonna strike again.'" I know a man who attributes his considerable success with women to the technique of being charming, attentive, and apparently completely impervious to each one.

Sexual pressure comes in an enormous variety of forms.

With strangers it ranges from the mild Christmas party ogle, through aggressive pickup lines, to direct physical assault. In many instances it is indistinguishable from sexual harassment. In the case of an established lover/husband, it sometimes takes the form of wheedling, which, as desperation grows, may descend into outright whining. But it is with a new date that women experience the most trying forms of pressure. There is no list long enough to include the variety of offenses that have been committed on such occasions. I can resort only to describing a few of the more common menaces.

Ex-Girlfriend Man: His previous girlfriend (he is quick to point out) was a Sex Goddess. He takes the new one out to dinner in an Indian restaurant. Halfway through the meal he slips his hands under her skirt and pretends that his fingers are a little man walking toward her panties. With chicken tikka masala poised between parted lips, she freezes. He looks surprised and says: "My ex-girlfriend used to love it when I did that."

On the walk back he tries again. He points at a muddy alley swarming with rats and muggers. "Let's go that way. No? Oh. My ex-girlfriend liked it up there. A great stargazer she was, if you get my meaning, ha, ha."

Back at his place, making out on the sofa, he muses that "my ex-girlfriend was real hot stuff" every time the woman shows reluctance to whip off her panties. Any woman fool enough to stick it out will discover that ex-girlfriend had long blond hair, a 36-24-35-inch figure, loved to prance naked around the room, and always had orgasms. When new woman decides she has to meet this marvel, it turns out she sailed last week for Venezuela.

Murmuring Man is more subtle. He entertains his date in near pitch-black: two flickering candles adorn the dinner table and the air is so thick with aftershave that a dew has accumulated on the walls. His conversation is devoted to how well he understands the female sex. "I lurve women," he breathes from out of the gloom. "I think you are getting excited about me, eh?"

Murmuring Man feeds a woman well: oysters mostly. Wine is uncorked and poured with a sequence of sidelong glances and a curious air of symbolism. As the clock ticks toward midnight he saunters to her side of the table, slides his hand around her waist, and murmurs, "Cummmun, Baby, I can tell you're dying for it."

She jumps up and screams.

All or Nothing Man is very different, being a true product of 1960s attitudes. He believes that any sort of sexual contact means you will thereafter automatically go all the way. He's usually young, and prides himself on having "no hang-ups." Any reluctance on the woman's part is interpreted as being "uptight." There's not a drop of humor to be gotten from him. "What's the matter with you? Are you frigid? Normal girls like fucking. That's what the sexual revolution was all about." She lies crumpled in the backseat of his car with the spotlight of freakishness glaring in her eyes. "It's not a good idea to cocktease a man," he advises.

It doesn't get any nicer if the girl gives in. Once he's got the promise of intercourse, this man's next move is to make the girl feel (as one woman interviewed by Shere Hite explained) "pressured into liking sex—being told that what feels good to him ought to be my primary satisfaction—if anal sex is a turn-on, a tight fit feels good, it's full speed ahead and damn the rectal fissures."

Sexual pressure is not flattering. It's exhausting. It's debasing. It is number one in women's list of turn-offs. Women know that men want to go to bed with them; they've been dealing with it since girlhood. If a man is too pushy it implies that he's simply in need of a lay, and there'll be little gratification in it for her.

"It's a rule," observes Jeanie, a forty-eight-year-old Liverpudlian, and one of only three women in an all-male office, "that the more a man pants the less involved you personally are. It's more a sense of 'Oh, any body will do.'" Sophistication, wit, intelligence, flattery, courtesy, respect, lack of sexual insistence— these are the ways to a woman's erotic heart, in no particular order, and preferably all rolled together.

Do Women Enjoy One-Night Stands?

In general, no. Occasionally, yes.

It's not the *briefness* of the encounter that turns women off, so much as the fact that men who go in for one-night stands tend to be unsympathetic. Many women have exquisite fantasies about meeting an attractive stranger for a single night of passion before kissing goodbye forever. But the stranger in the fantasy always knows what he's about, and the pleasure is mutual. In real life, a woman runs a high risk of picking a dud. If every decent, sensitive, sexually educated man with an attractive penis were marked with a red beacon, the number of one-night stands would increase dramatically. "Women are equally interested initially," wrote one reader, "but lack of proper stimulation, orgasm, and quick uncaring lovers gradually makes women feel like sex is something that men enjoy more."

Sex with an unfamiliar man is risky. If it goes wrong, women have a lot to lose. Quite apart from his quality as a lover, every time she gets involved she has to consider four things: Is he violent? Is he diseased? Will I get pregnant? What will this do to my reputation? These color a woman's attitude to sex—casual sex in particular—so deeply that they are worth looking at in more detail.

Violence: Male violence is never far from a woman's thoughts. It is random, commonplace, and by no means confined to thugs with broken noses and tattoos on their foreheads. Sandra Horley, director of a women's shelter, picks out a common type of culprit whom she calls Charm Syndrome Man: "What these men have in common is that they are invariably the last people anyone would suspect of abusing their partners." They "present a likable face to the rest of the world: charm obscures the abuser."

At least one-third of women have endured some form of sexual violence. The real figure is probably higher. Most abusers are men known to the women, and many attacks happen in nonsexual situations. Not surprisingly, they often permanently scar the woman's attitude to men and sex.

Disease: Women can readily pick up sexually transmitted diseases, because an infected man deposits his infected fluid inside her body. AIDS is the big one, of course. Intravenous drug users, men who've had blood transfusions, bisexuals, men who've been to prostitutes—a large section of the male population is in the high risk category for HIV infection. No one knows how widespread the illness is. Then there's syphilis, gonorrhea, and a host of other, more minor pleasantries. A woman has to consider not only how these will affect her, but how they will affect the health of any children she might have in the future.

Pregnancy: In the middle of sex, it'll sometimes dawn on a woman that between her and motherhood is a fraction of a millimeter of rubber famous for its liability to break, or a diaphragm known for its tendency to slip out of place. Contraceptives are fallible. Every time she has intercourse a woman runs the risk of nine months of feeling awful, losing her job, and being lumbered with a demanding new creature who'll be with her for the next twenty years. Alternatively, she can have a highly traumatic abortion (*if* she can get one).

Reputation: Old-fashioned though this may sound, our society has not come to terms with women's sexuality. For all the so-called liberation, the sexual double standard still does a great

deal to stifle women's sex drive. At school, it is a favorite pastime of pubescent boys to call girls who don't go far enough ice
queens, and those who do, whores. This attitude is by no
means confined to schoolkids:

> Sexual women are still treated with suspicion by a lot
> of people, especially the older generation. It isn't just a
> happy fling for them. It's the possibility of a look in the
> office. Parents' snide remarks. Feeling that you're avail-
> able to anyone who hears about your activities. Women
> have to tread carefully. Who is the man behind the
> penis? Sex can be dangerous to the body and the repu-
> tation.

A lot of women have had very sad experiences of casual
sex, and went out of their way to counsel other women not to
repeat their mistakes:

> Be yourself, relax, enjoy and don't ever rush yourself.
> Get to know your mate, don't ever jump in bed with a
> stranger, he is not gonna call or come back and he is
> only after what he can get. Find someone and get to
> know him, then enjoy.

Ultimately, of course, there's no way of telling whether a
woman's going to be interested in casual sex or not until she
actually makes her desires clear. Most women say they'd prefer
to have sex with a man they love but, failing that, any good
lover will do. The London tabloid *Mail on Sunday* conducted a
poll in 1993 and found that more than a third of women said
they would get into bed with a new partner simply for the sex,
with no strings attached, although they wanted time to get to
know him first. Quilliam, on the other hand, found that over
half of her women would have intercourse on a first date, if the
circumstances were right.

Getting a woman drunk is not considered a popular approach. Most women feel tacky the next day when their one-night stand was alcohol-inspired, and often downright furious. One-night stands inspired purely by lust, on the other hand, are popular and seldom regretted. To women brought up believing sex was only proper with commitment, this comes as a nice surprise. "I thought it could never happen to me that I could be with someone for one night, enjoy it, and just forget about it," says Beatrice Aristimuno, a fashion editor and public relations whatsit. "Well, it did happen, and I didn't feel a shit, I didn't feel a whore . . . I just felt great."

Erica Jong calls the ideal brief encounter a "zipless fuck," in which the sex is totally uncomplicated. I know only one woman who's ever had one (she's a high-powered lawyer now) and she enjoyed it enormously. The setting was, oddly, very similar to the one Jong describes in her book. She was about twenty-two years old and traveling across Switzerland by train. She hadn't booked a sleeper and so was sitting in a cabin with seven other people, and next to an extremely attractive man. At ten o'clock the guard came around and distributed blankets, which they spread over their laps. The guard left and the lights were dimmed; underneath the blanket the attractive man's hand reached over and touched hers. She unzipped his pants; he parted her legs. They spent the night satisfying each other beneath the blanket in the presence of all the others. Early in the morning my friend got off at her station without ever having spoken a word to the pleasant young man.

Women Like Seducing Men

"Her insistence on sexual contact was extremely embarrassing," recalled Robert Yerkes. "Throwing herself on her back she pressed herself against my feet and repeatedly and determinedly tried to pull me upon her . . . She was markedly and vigorously aggressive, and it required considerable adroitness and strength of resistance on my part to withstand her attack . . . [She was] determined in her efforts to satisfy her desire."

The seductress was Congo, a female gorilla. Dr. Yerkes was lucky to get away with his life. Most men, however, are absolutely delighted to be ravished by a female. And most women, once they pluck up courage to do it, find being in control of the evening exhilarating and very sexy. This is not the least of the reasons why pressure from men is so unsexy—it never gives us a chance!

It is certainly not innate in women to be the less forward partner. In numerous cultures outside of our own, women are expected to make the sexual advances. At a ceremonial dance in Colombia, a Gaojiro Indian woman who fancies a man must try to trip him up. If she succeeds, he is duty-bound to have sex with her. The thoroughly modern Lolicia declares, "I was never seduced. I always seduced everybody. Nobody ever seduced me." I also dislike the role of seducee, and I believe passionately that the more sexual initiative women take, the better for everybody.

Women who feel in control in the bedroom—not "prey"—have a greater chance of orgasm. Seduction gives women confidence and men a much needed break from the anxieties of always making the first move.

> I find it extremely sexy when a woman opens a door for me—it's exhausting to always have to be the one to do the little courtesies, to remember to be "attentive," or romantic.
>
> Last year a woman in my office, a year or two older than me but much junior in status, whom I'd never paid the slightest attention to before, came up to me and fanned two theater tickets in front of my nose. I was so surprised I just said yes. She wasn't much to look at but I was intrigued by her chutzpah. She said she'd pick me

up: she turned up in a battered green open-topped MG, very cool. She took everything in hand. I had five minutes of feeling my manhood was at stake—then swooned into the evening. God bless women's liberation! —Gary

Romance? Leave it to the girls. Look, I'm forty-eight. It's pure bliss to give the girls a turn. Why not? Women are tougher than men, why should we coddle them, and make them feel they have to be petted and fussed over like halfwits? Nobody enjoys it. —Robert

When I first meet a woman I have what I call a "putting out the feelers" period. I try to figure out whether she's going to be the type to take the lead, or prefers it to be me. I don't mind which way it is—but I enjoy the fact that it can be both. —Oliver

Women are rapidly discovering the delights of making the first move: "Take a situation that happened to me the other week," explains Winny, twenty-seven. "On the bus I started talking to a man I liked the look of and ended up going out to supper with him and taking him home, where we made love in front of the fire. It was beautiful. He was great. I wasn't worried about 'giving myself' and didn't feel exploited when I sucked him or guilty when he went down on me. It was a sudden burst of lust and that was it. I felt it and indulged it and after three hours I was totally exhausted and we slept naked on the rug by the fire until dawn. I'm totally relaxed about it. Now that never would have been possible in my mother's day, which is why she's so screwed up about sex and why my father said all women were whores or frigid."

I want a man to show interest and then it's my turn, back and forth until we end up in a relationship and then into bed. I want the heat to come from him and I reflect it back. If I have to make the first move then he damn well better jump—I mean find a way to let me know it's what he wants . . . no one wants to feel pushed or manipulated.

My rule is: if he waits for me, then I'm interested. If I want the guy then, I'll make it clear. I can't stand the pushy, fuck-me, feel-my-prick type. I like the dalliance. It makes the first night in bed much sexier. I like a man to play the game.

I personally have sent the shyest of men wild by seducing them.

Every single reader whom I questioned said that sex was better for both partners if women were *not* submissive—unless it was part of role-playing.

A man admires and finds it sexy to make love to a woman who is aware of her sexual needs and has no problem in asserting her force. I think they feel flattered.

There are some rare cases—those men who don't like women initiating sex—but those men aren't worth the trouble anyway. I feel very strongly about that.

Except for the first man I ever slept with . . . I was the one to initiate it, and they all seemed relieved. I threw the ball out and we played a good game. A woman should only be submissive if it's some sort of role-playing, fantasy situation. Men don't like a woman who just lies there. I've asked.

This attitude is reflected in what women find erotic in stories and on film. In a study published in the *Journal of Sex Research,* women said that erotic stories in which the female was the dominant partner were much more exciting than when it was the other way around. Books in which the woman is submissive provide "the kind of context which females find the least arousing and which elicits more negative effect."

The great majority of men find the idea of women taking command extremely sexy. But women still hold back: they fear being thought "pushy" or "unfeminine." So, male readers, take every opportunity to impress on women that men like them to make the first move. Tell not just girlfriends, but all the women you meet.

Why Don't More Women Use Male Prostitutes?

For a woman in need of casual, uncomplicated sex, you'd think that male prostitutes would be popular. A gigolo should satisfy all the requirements for a good fling, after all. He's physically attractive and probably good in bed. He's unlikely to be violent, and a woman could easily confine herself only to those who were sterilized and with certificates of good health. By using a whorehouse outside the locality she could safeguard her reputation as well.

Yet male brothels aren't popular. In 1995, a set of store-fronted rooms opened in Amsterdam, each with an attractive man plus bed. Women, it was hoped, would come along, inspect the goods on offer, and then use whichever one took their fancy. The experiment was short-lived and most of the customers were local prostitutes!

The reason, once again, has to do with context. Many more women would be interested in paying for good sex if it was managed in the right way. But instead of setting up something specifically for women, the Dutch entrepreneurs simply produced a string of brothels of the sort men like, and changed the sex of the prostitutes.

I've often thought about opening a women's brothel myself.

The initial appointment would be made by telephone, during which the client would chat to the men available and eliminate the no-hopers. (The telephone is an excellent medium for testing a man's attractiveness.) Next she would show up at the house and meet her shortlist, all of them fully clothed. Their looks should be varied. An endless stream of rock-jawed male models, such as the sort who appear in women's magazines advertising perfume, would be tedious. I'd employ some tall slender ones, a couple of short chunkies, a beefy hunk, and of course a range of "looks"—studious, athletic, super-stylish, etc. After half an hour spent in company of the shortlist, the client makes her choice, and they leave together. Just as men's brothels cater to different forms of kinkiness, women's brothels should provide for different types of context. Now they would spend several hours larking around doing whatever activity the client chooses—it could be anything from an evening at the opera, a rave party, or watching dirty films in Times Square, to an afternoon's sailing followed by a visit to the Met. She may lure him into bed at any time—or never. There is no obligation for sex at all.

A woman's brothel is halfway between an escort agency and a traditional whorehouse. The client doesn't have to provide the premises and gets to look over the goods, but she also gets to take her choice away on loan in order to get the circumstances of the sex right. Prices would start at $50 an hour.

Nearly two hundred years ago one Mary Wilson had a similar idea to mine, described in her erotic book *The Voluptuarian Cabinet* of 1824. She has, she says, purchased very extensive premises, elegantly and commodiously fitted up with erotic paintings and exquisite food and drink. The lady clients (many married) remain blissfully anonymous by wearing masks:

> In these saloons, according to their classes, are to be seen the finest men of their species I can procure, occupied in whatever amusements are adapted to their

taste, and all kept in a state of high excitement by good living and idleness. The ladies will never enter the saloons even in their masks, but view their inmates from a darkened window in each boudoir. In one they will see fine, elegantly dressed young men playing cards, music, &c.—in others athletic men wrestling or bathing, in a state of perfect nudity. In short, they will see such a variety of the animal that they cannot fail of suiting their inclinations. Having fixed upon one she should like to enjoy, the lady has only to ring for the chambermaid, call her to the window, point out the object, and he is immediately brought to the boudoir. She can enjoy him in the dark, or have a light and keep on her mask. She can stay for an hour or a night, and have one or a dozen men as she pleases, without being known to any of them . . . The whole expense of the Institution is defrayed by a subscription from each lady of one hundred guineas per annum.

The Questionnaire

I would very much like to know more of my readers' opinions and experiences of sex. The more information that is exchanged, the better able men and women are to please each other. Your replies will be treated in strict confidence. There is no need to supply a name or address, but other details about yourself are very welcome—your age, job, background, etc., and most important of all, whether you are a man or a woman! Please feel free to write as fully as you like: stories, experiences, and strongly held opinions are particularly helpful. If you are very busy, just choose the questions that interest you. I would much rather you answered a few in detail than all of them briefly.

The completed questionnaire should be sent to me, via the publisher (all letters are forwarded without being opened).

Please be honest in your answers.

Questionnaire for Men

Men and Women

1. Describe your ideal woman.

2. What first attracts you to a woman?

3. Can you list the qualities that you believe essential to your being attracted to a woman? If you are easygoing on this matter, please say so.

4. What do you like least about women?

5. Do you feel that greater equality of the sexes has improved the quality of your life? Or would you prefer it if women behaved more as they did twenty or thirty years ago?

6. Do you find women who dress in an obviously sexy manner—short skirt, cleavage, etc.—more alluring or less?

7. Who (among well-known people) is your idea of a really good-looking woman?

8. Which well-known woman would you most like to be married to, and why?

9. What do you think of when you hear the word "feminist"?

10. Do you find working together with a woman more likely or less likely to lead to you finding her attractive?

11. Who do you consider a good role model for women?

12. Are you happy with your own looks? If not, why not?

13. Have you ever had cosmetic surgery? If not, would you ever consider it, and what sort?

14. Who (among well-known people) is your idea of a really good-looking man?

15. Who among well-known men would you like to change places with?

16. What quality do you most dislike in other men?

17. What *in your experience* do you think women notice in a man?

18. Who do you consider a good role model for men?

Quality of Sex

19. On a scale of 1 (lowest) to 10 (highest), how good is sex, on average? How often is it 10? How often is it 1?

20. Do you ever think other people have more exciting sex lives than you do?

21. When sex is disappointing, what has made it so?

22. Is there any particular thing that you find women are reluctant to do in bed?

23. Is your current partner willing to do what you want in bed?

24. What, in your experience, do most women do wrong in bed?

25. Do you prefer a passive or an active sexual partner, or a mixture of the two?

26. What are your views on going to bed with a virgin? Would it excite you, worry you, or neither?

27. What is your favorite sexual position?

28. Do women usually perform oral sex (a) willingly (b) well?

29. Do women usually perform manual sex (a) willingly (b) well?

30. Where do you normally have sex?

31. Have you ever been caught by a third person in the middle of making love?

32. How long does sex usually last for you?

33. What aspects of sex are likely to make you come quicker or come slower?

34. Do women complain much in bed, or do you find they usually appear happy with the lovemaking?

35. What do you like a woman to wear in bed?

Hot Stuff

36. If you had a sex slave, what would you have her do to you?

37. And what would you do to her?

38. Have you ever acted out your fantasies? Was it worth it?

39. Have you ever had homosexual fantasies?

40. Have you ever had fantasies of doing sexually illegal things?

41. Have you ever had sex with more than one partner? Can you give details?

42. If you *had* to admit to a "fetish," what would yours be?

43. What is the most unusual place you've ever made love?

44. Have you ever had sex with an older woman? If so, how much older was she?

45. Can you say how satisfactory the sex was?

46. Do you find unusual sexual positions enjoyable?

47. What is the single sexiest moment you can ever remember? It need not be a whole night, or even involve full sex, but something that sticks in your mind as exceptionally arousing.

48. What is the most sexually adventurous thing you have ever done?

Satisfaction

49. Have you ever faked an orgasm? How? Did you get away with it?

50. Have you ever had multiple orgasms? Did you teach yourself to do it, or did it happen naturally?

51. Chapter 13 contains the Multiple Orgasm Plan for men. If you have tried it, can you give any information about your success?

52. In your experience, do women want orgasms?

Infidelity

53. Have you ever been unfaithful? If yes, does this happen often?

54. Did/do you regret it?

55. Was it worth being unfaithful—did the sex live up to it?

56. What would you do if you found your partner was unfaithful? Would it end the relationship?

57. Do you think men or women are more prone to infidelity?

Sexual Parts

58. Do you find women's genitals attractive?

59. Do you enjoy performing oral sex on a woman?

60. If no to either question, why not?

61. In your experience, do women enjoy having oral sex performed on them?

62. Have you ever suffered inability to get an erection? Explain the circumstances and how (if) it was cured.

63. Are you circumcised?

64. Are you happy with your own penis?

65. If you could change one aspect of it, what would it be?

66. Has any woman ever made a comment about your penis?

67. Do you think women prefer a large penis?

68. How large is your penis?

69. Have you any sex tips or experiences that you would like to tell? Or anything else on the subject of women and sex?

Questionnaire for Women

Men and Women

1. Describe your ideal man.

2. What first attracts you to a man?

3. Can you list the qualities that you believe essential to your being attracted to a man? If you are easygoing on this matter, please say so.

4. What do you like least about men?

5. Do you feel that greater equality of the sexes has improved the quality of your life? Or would you prefer it if women and/or men behaved more as they did twenty or thirty years ago?

6. Do you find very obviously good-looking men attractive, or are you wary of them?

7. Who (among well-known people) is your idea of a really good-looking man?

8. Which well-known man would you most like to be married to, and why?

9. What do you think of when you hear the word "feminist"?

10. Do you find working together with a man more likely or less likely to lead to you finding him attractive?

11. Who do you consider a good role model for men?

12. Are you happy with your own looks? If not, why not?

13. Have you ever had cosmetic surgery? If not, would you ever consider it, and what sort?

14. Who (among well-known people) is your idea of a really good-looking woman?

15. Who among well-known women would you like to change places with?

16. What quality do you most dislike in other women?

17. What *in your experience* do you think men notice in a woman?

18. Who do you consider a good role model for women?

Quality of Sex

19. On a scale of 1 (lowest) to 10 (highest), how good is sex, on average? How often is it 10? How often is it 1?

20. Do you ever think other people have more exciting sex lives than you do?

21. When sex is disappointing, what has made it so?

22. Is there any particular thing that you find men are reluctant to do in bed?

23. Is your current partner willing to do what you want in bed?

24. What, in your experience, do most men do wrong in bed?

25. Do you like a man to take the initiative in bed, or for him to be more passive?

26. What are your views on going to bed with a virgin? Would it excite you, worry you, or neither?

27. What is your favorite sexual position?

28. Do men usually perform oral sex (a) willingly (b) well?

29. Do men usually perform manual sex (a) willingly (b) well?

30. Where do you normally have sex?

31. Have you ever been caught by a third person in the middle of making love?

32. How long would you like sex to last ideally?

33. What aspects of sex are most important to enable you to reach orgasm, or get as close as you do?

34. Are men too demanding in their lovemaking? For example, do they too often expect women to change position or experiment?

35. What do you like a man to wear in bed?

Hot Stuff

36. If you had a sex slave, what would you have him do to you?

37. And what would you do to him?

38. Have you ever acted out your fantasies? Was it worth it?

39. Have you ever had lesbian fantasies?

40. Have you ever had fantasies of doing sexually illegal things?

41. Have you ever had sex with more than one partner? Can you give details?

42. If you *had* to admit to a "fetish," what would yours be?

43. What is the most unusual place you've ever made love?

44. Have you ever had sex with a younger man? If so, how much younger was he?

45. Can you say how satisfactory the sex was?

46. Do you find unusual sexual positions enjoyable?

47. What is the single sexiest moment you can ever remember? It need not be a whole night, or even involve full sex, but something that sticks in your mind as exceptionally arousing.

48. What is the most sexually adventurous thing you have ever done?

Satisfaction

49. Have you ever faked an orgasm? How? Did you get away with it?

50. Have you ever had multiple orgasms? By that I mean not just several in one session, but several in a row with only a few seconds' gap. Did you teach yourself to do it, or did it happen naturally?

51. What is the greatest sexual ability that you have come across in a man?

52. How important is orgasm for you?

Infidelity

53. Have you ever been unfaithful? If yes, does this happen often?

54. Did/do you regret it?

55. Was it worth being unfaithful—did the sex live up to it?

56. What would you do if you found your partner was unfaithful? Would it end the relationship?

57. Do you think men or women are more prone to infidelity?

Sexual Parts

58. Do you find men's genitals attractive?

59. Do you enjoy performing oral sex on a man?

60. If no to either question, why not?

61. What percentage of men perform oral sex with real skill?

62. Has a partner of yours ever suffered inability to get an erection? Explain the circumstances and how (if) it was cured. Were you upset by it, or philosophical?

63. Were most of the men you have been to bed with circumcised or uncircumcised?

64. Describe your ideal penis.

65. Is it important to you how a man's body looks? For example, if he was nice could you want him regardless of his shape?

66. Could you ever be turned off by the look of a man's penis?

67. Do you enjoy penetration?

68. What is your opinion of anal sex?

69. Have you any sex tips or experiences that you would like to tell? Or anything else on the subject of women and sex?

3

What Drives Women Wild?

*T*hink you know the answer? Forget it! The biggest difference of all between women and men comes in the way
they answer this question. Men, for example, invariably put
broad chest, sturdy shoulders, and pumped-up biceps on top
of the list, which is why otherwise quite sensible individuals go
to gyms, dislocate their backs trying to lift a ton and a half of
metal slabs, and have conversations of the following type,
recorded verbatim at my local bar, during a particularly bad
Muscle Man infestation:

Muscle Man One (*displaying enormous biceps*): Feel
that. Rock hard, that is.

Muscle Man Two: Peanuts!

MM One: Smash your nose, it would.

MM Two: No chance.

MM One: Show us what you got then.

MM Two (*rolls up sleeve to reveal enormous flexed
muscle*): That's iron. Lay you flat in no time.

MM One (*feeling the item in question*): Soft as jelly. Etc.

The women sitting next to these two were certainly driven wild—with hysterical laughter. Yet Muscle Men persist in their conviction that women want to be carried off into the trees, Johnny Weissmuller fashion. Even my lean-bean boyfriend informs me that Muscle Man is part of most men's psyche, his own included, as he sheepishly admitted. I stared in disbelief. "It's part of being masculine," he explained. "You don't have to *be* muscly, but you have to *think* muscly. You've got to know of at least one or two positions in which you're not an absolute reed. Poses you can practice in front of the mirror and adopt at the swimming pool. Keeping your arms squeezed tight against your side, so that whenever you bend them the biceps appear larger is a good trick. It's mental too. Think strong. Think manly."

Yet most women couldn't give a hoot about men's muscles. It's not the monsters with chests like Mount Vesuvius and arms whose veins have emigrated to the outer skin layer who are admired. Women like bottoms.

The defining characteristics of a good bottom are the same ones as for a miser: small, tight, and narrow. One should be able to hold each buttock in the grasp of a woman's hand, since such like clutching is, from our point of view, the chief use of a man's bottom during sex. Nothing so off-putting in a passionate moment as grasping a flabby bottom.

If I had to choose a physical factor it would have to be a man's butt. It's his most private part, in a way. I like a tall, dark man. Italian. Intellectual. His body's got to be attractive, but slender. Proportions matter much more than muscle, which is, let's face it, not all that interesting. Gay magazine stuff.

Women have an intimate relationship with male bottoms. During sex, it's the part we touch most. If we control its move-

What men imagine women admire (percent)		What women really admire (percent)
Tallness 13		Tallness 5
Hair—texture, not length 4		Hair—texture, not length 5
Eyes..............................4		Eyes.............................11
Neck.............................2		Neck.............................3
Muscular chest and shoulders...........21		Muscular chest and shoulders..............1
Muscular arms 18		Muscular arms 0
Slimness 7		Slimness 15
Flat stomach 9		Flat stomach..............13
Buttocks......................4		Buttocks—described as small and sexy.....39
Large penis 15		Penis............................2
Long legs 3		Long legs 6

What men think women admire in a man, and what we actually do admire. Taken from Luria et al., *Human Sexuality.*

ment, we control the pace of intercourse and the area of strongest stimulation between our legs—both of which are vitally important for female sexual satisfaction. A top-notch bottom should give no hint of a feminine curve. Former British prime minister John Major's, for example, is not a choice specimen. It is a typical postwar British bottom, the sort that makes the tails of a jacket split apart and the waist crumple upward.

Next on many women's list is slimness, particularly a flat stomach. Men look much worse than women when they're overweight. Well-padded women can look curvy and delicious, and the weight is more evenly spread. Men simply look as if their chest has slipped. I support my fellow females on this point absolutely: my ideal man is so lean he has to run around in the shower to get wet. On the beach the guy I notice is not the hulking brute in the much-too-revealing-to-be-sexy swimming trunks, but the mild fellow minding his own business who gets sand kicked in his face. It brings out all my chivalrous instincts and I plot how to seduce him on the spot.

After pretty bottoms and slenderness, it's eyes:

> Once had a fling with a man I met (eyes are the best for me) and he had black eyes and long eyelashes. It turned me wild. He was quite short. Saw him on the subway and followed him home because I had to find out where he lived. Lucky! On his own. I didn't mind what he did. I wanted to look in his eyes as he did it. Once he masturbated me when we were having supper at a French restaurant. I did it to him too. Watching him come and try to control his face was the most ecstatic thing I've ever done. His eyes looked incredibly worried but he couldn't stop. Mmmmmmmmmm!

Paul Newman blue eyes will secure success whatever your shape. It is not just the color that matters, but the expression. Determined, steely eyes in the Clint Eastwood mold are good from time to time, but usually much less effective than sensitive eyes. Sexy eyes should convey excitement, responsiveness, humor, intelligence. "I could not fancy him," declared Renate, a sultry Viennese, of a good-looking admirer. "His eyes are dull, no sparkle, no intelligence. Without that even the most handsome man's face is dull. I say to myself, 'This is a dull man.'"

After these three essentials it's a free-for-all. One woman's dish is another's poison. Tall, short, bald, mophead, dark, light, clean-shaven, fuzzy, they've all got their adherents:

> Working in the health and fitness trade I obviously see a lot of good bodies. In terms of beauty of body I would put the male athletes in the following order: middle distance, sprinters, swimmers. Marathoners are

too skinny. Weight lifters turn me right off. Dancers, when I get them, are lovely.

Part of the reason I came to Göttingen, Germany, is because I love the academic look in a man. I find the innocent, preoccupied look very attractive. I can't bear sporty types. It's an intelligence thing, I think. I've noticed that most of my intelligent, self-confident friends feel the same.

Japanese men don't have a reputation in England for being handsome, but modern Japan is full of tall, dark, and gorgeous young men. Best of all, they have silky smooth skin. I hate body hair.

I like a man to have a V-shaped torso with a hairy chest. Not a gladiator, but lean and fit-looking, with a tan. A man's got to be strong, masculine.

A Regency dandy is my wow. Somebody with grace and style. Foppish.

One of the most important features of my own Mr. Right is a large nose, not because it promises large sexual equipment (hands and feet are better indicators of that) but because it gives his face authority and distinction. He's terribly English and reserved, spends his spare time improving Einstein's theory of general relativity, and is as pale as an aspirin tablet. I am unusual, however. The majority of women seem to go crazy for the Italianate types, because of the dark complexion and their reputation for being sophisticated, attentive lovers.

Condolences were offered to me on two occasions on account of my pallor, and Jaua was probably expressing the opinion of the majority when he said that if he were white he supposed that he, too, would be ashamed and cover his body with as many clothes as possible.

—DR. HOGBIN, AMONG THE NATIVES OF
WOGEO, NEW GUINEA

The thing that really drives women wild with disgust is dirty men. This, according to anthropologists and Swift readers alike, is universal.

> Yuck! Socks. Smelly socks. Turns you off a man. Dirty hands and fingernails, ditto. Just couldn't have sex with him. Men who come to bed reeking of their job—oil, lubricant and all that. Men who don't wash their genitals—so you're all sexy, warm and waiting for a good time—then *phew!* Not bothering to wash tells me: "You're not worth the trouble" or "I don't think about you." A man goes inside a woman. I don't want all that muck inside me!

> Nose hair is disgusting. Ear hair—pretty bad. Bad shaving: makes a man look like a grubby carpet.

A man has two lines of attack when it comes to driving a woman wild with desire: his body and his other parts. Women are much more interested in the other parts than men imagine. Sexiness might have nothing to do with a man's physical qualities at all:

> The most attractive man I've met recently wasn't that much in the physical stakes. I met him in the library. It was hot summer. I was bored and sick of satisfying myself underneath the table. I came back to my table and found a note there.
>   "Zaftig and eesome, tretis as Venus, I love you completely."

As you know, I'm a bit of a logophile myself, so this note stuck a chord. Zaftig I knew, and it was true I was on the plump side. Tretis I wasn't sure of, but I felt it must have been flattering if Venus possessed it. I looked around and saw a middle-aged, not too unserviceable man with nice glasses watching me. I was really turned on by his approach.

I decided it was bluntness or nothing:

"Leptosome lover, engage in syndyasmian pleasure with your bustluscious and callipygian nymph."

In short, I took him in the restroom.

The difficulty: sweet as he was as a logophile, he suffered from severe tachorgasmia. Serious meupareunia. Look those ones up yourself!

Even an ugly toad can do well if he's sufficiently endowed in the abstract department: Sartre (brains), Onassis (wealth), Rasputin (hypnotism) are all examples of this. Women's capacity to fall for peculiar-looking individuals is famous—"Why fat men are attractive," cry the women's glossies, "Why bald men are sexy," "Why short men are the best lovers," and, yes, even this one has seen the light of day: "Why ugly men turn me on." The explanation offered for this willful behavior is almost always to do with the stereotypical personality of such men, rather than their distinguishing physical features. As Shirley MacLaine put it: "It's always the mind with me. I don't care if the guy looks like a bowling ball." Professionalism, for example, is an extremely powerful aphrodisiac for women: from bricklayer to president, a man who does something with great skill and control will usually have the edge over a better-looking bungler. It is one reason why so many women fall in love with their doctor, or their vet, or their driving instructor. But it must be effortless ability, not puffed-up boastfulness.

There is one abstract feature that invariably comes top of

every poll on the subject. Just cast your eye down the lonely hearts columns: GSOH.

GSOH? It took me ages to work it out the first time I came across it. Gorgeous, Sexy, Oriental Hominid? Gottahave Sex Outside House (i.e., I have wife and two kids, so no romps at home)? But in that case, why should a DJMNSNR "artist" with MBA, seeking SJPW, also want GSOH (RSVP)? I mean, he said he was D, didn't he?

Women have a weakness for men who make them laugh. "It's the best aphrodisiac going. Humor gives me an orgasm much quicker than a big prick," remarks Sondra. "Funny men, men who are interested in what I do, men who talk well . . . I like a man who's good company, whether by way of his humor or his intelligence." Although, as a handsome young woman I was speaking to in a store remarked, "it's extremely suspicious that these people all need to advertise their GSOH. A sense of humor is so essential to any decent human being that I'd be inclined to give him a miss. I'd be happier with someone who took their sense of humor for granted—or perhaps someone who advertised BSOH or NSOH."

Why is humor so important to us? Men also like it in their partners, but it's not as sought after as it is by women. Some females are prepared to give up almost everything else in its honor. The main reason is that it reduces sexual pressure. Humor is one of the few ways a woman can feel at ease with a man—particularly an unfamiliar, eligible man—without sex immediately becoming an issue. Humor is relaxing, yet at the same time it can be extremely intimate, "because," explains my psychologist friend, "it forces a person to laugh even against her will, as if the man who's made her laugh has managed to break down all her defenses. An intimate relationship with a man like this will not be centered entirely around the bedroom." Interestingly, the one time when humor is considered a turn-off is when it's overtly sexual. Women hate explicit sexual witticism from men they don't know well.

Joke-telling and humor are not the same thing, however. Every woman dreads being cornered by:

Monty Python Man: The impersonator. The rib digger. He can recite the dead parrot sketch word perfect, and when he gets to the *Fawlty Towers* hamster-that-was-really-a-rat he does the voices too. Jokes are his forte—he's always loved a good 'un. He's a man who never lets a minute pass without extending it to two minutes with an invigorating witticism. When his memory's exhausted he turns to his copy of *More Hockey Jokes*. The triumph of the evening is when he leaps up from the barstool and struts across the room popping his neck in and out like a chicken.

"Humor is being able to laugh at yourself, or see absurdity in small situations. Not caper about with a paper bag on your head," remarks Geraldine (who had to endure just that).

Francie sees humor as sharing: "All my life I've gone for men who make it clear they want to share life with me. I don't want a total comedian. I had one of those once and it was laugh all day long until my sides split, but it was always him making the jokes. Whenever I ventured one, it was silence. Okay, I tell bad jokes. I felt outside him, though. I was always an audience with Tom. It was exhausting."

One of women's *greatest* frustrations is that too few men take the trouble to listen, ask, or draw them out about their activities and opinions. It is the cause of innumerable divorces and one of the main reasons women, in desperation, turn to other men. "He listened to me" . . . "I became an individual again, not an adjunct to him" . . . "I felt steamrollered by my husband," etc., etc., etc., are much more common explanations for infidelity than "he had thirty-inch biceps, a face like Tom Cruise, and a whopping great willy." For many women the only talk about their own concerns they get from their man is a lecture—a lengthy monologue on what she is doing wrong/right and how she ought to improve her position by doing this, that, or the other. In fact I was much amused to read recently that studies have shown that men nowadays nag *more* than women!

It is not strictly true that **Monologue Man** drives women wild, he anesthetizes them. Once such a character gets going, he's *interminable!* He babbles for hours; his date puts in fifteen seconds; he talks for another forty minutes; she squeezes in fifty-nine seconds; he comes away complaining how women chatter. The world's myriad victims of Monologue Man will tell you that the idea that women are the babbling sex is nothing more than prejudice and the fact that our higher voices are more noticeable than men's. (In a study published in *Psychology Today,* teachers were shown a film of classroom discussions and asked which sex was talking more. Overwhelmingly, they said the girls were. Actually the boys were talking *three times* as much.)

Monologue Man comes in a wide variety of types, from the pompous professional to the nineteen-year-old student whom Carolyn went out with in her first year at college:

> He began the moment he picked me up at the college gates, making comparisons either explicit or tacit. "I drank that amazing number of pints, was sick in these various places, was defiant to this, that and the other person, and by the way, since I'm leaning towards you in this completely admirable and sexually inspiring fashion, haven't you noticed that my shoulders are bigger than everybody else's in the room?" and so on . . . Always trying to impress me. He couldn't see that the only way I'd be impressed was if he showed a little modesty about himself.

As the novelist Kate Chopin so nicely puts it: "Robert talked a good deal about himself. He was very young, and did not know any better."

Two further specimens of Monologue Man are particularly familiar to women:

Restaurant Man appreciates the finer things in life. He knows about food. "Quite a good little place we're going to tonight," he throws out casually. "So dress the part, eh?"

The restaurant is not half as grand as he implied. His woman guest/victim feels hideously overdressed. Restaurant Man begins as he'll go on—by twirling a thimbleful of wine in his glass, snorting up the fumes with a great, connoisseurial sigh, and exclaiming:

"Unexceptable. Couldn't possibly drink it."

The moules marinière are a touch too salty. The boeuf bourguignon is superb; he must congratulate the chef. The crème brulée has been baked in piss.

By the end of the evening his escort has shrunk to half her height. The other half is under the table. He still hasn't registered that she's not a librarian, and calls her Di even though she's said a hundred times that her name's Diana. Restaurant Man makes a point of leaving a tip to match the quality of the service (7½ percent).

Museum Man is the monster of the museum and art gallery circuit. The fellow who hurries ahead to each exhibit, reads the labels, then returns to his dutiful wife and children to explain in a loud voice what it's all about. In advanced cases, he'll provide an analysis of the relic/painting/tapestry, punctuating his monologue with remarks such as "It is interesting to note that" and "I'm of the opinion." In the absence of a label, he complains about the degeneracy of learning and says he will write a letter to the director "forthwith." His wife is permanently hot from blushing. The children are maladjusted. In my experience, this man is often bearded.

Beside men such as these—men who, I believe, consider themselves instructive, informative, admirable, manly, and endowed with the essential qualities of leadership—women feel a lack of existence. The most attractive male is the one who listens, shares his feelings, acknowledges his weaknesses, expresses his doubts, and shows as much concern for the woman's affairs as for his own. *I cannot overstress how often women say this.* It applies not just to lovers, but to all relationships with men. Real estate agents, for example, have little idea of how much business they lose by talking down to prospective women clients. When I put my extremely desirable residence on the market recently, six of them vied for the commission, and I chose the only one who didn't try to patronize me. Like an increasing number of other women, I like a female accountant and a female bank manager, not because I think women are better at these jobs, but because experience has shown me that professional women are less likely to waste my time being all-knowing, "manly," and pompous. They listen more and admit mistakes instead of trying to cover up with bluster or blame their secretary.

"A seductive man listens," writes Grace, thirty-six, from Atlanta. "He is a friend and companion. He shares his time with a woman. Timothy was like that from the start. I knew he was the one for me because I felt we were equal when we talked. I forgot about everyone else and spent the whole night laughing and arguing. We didn't get around to the sex until the middle of the next day. It was a natural progression."

> Not listening to what I have to say is a bad sign in a prospective lover. A person who over- and out-talks everybody else is nine times out of ten bad in bed. If he can't even manage to be unselfish in conversation, then he's not going to become suddenly altruistic when the lights are off.

> My golden advice to any man trying to pick up a woman is: don't lecture and don't attempt to pull the

world-adventurer, brave-as-a-lion, intellectual genius stunt either. It's a loser. Get a conversation going in which the topic is shared by you and the woman. Seduce her by making her feel comfortable.

—A. H. ["one who knows"], London

"Macho Does Not Prove Mucho"
—Zsa Zsa Gabor

Ninety percent of women are feminists. They may hate the word but they fully support the basic principles of the movement, that women and men should have equal consideration in law, in politics, at work, at home, in bed. "It's amazing," exclaims Dr. M. S., from London, "all my female students' essays are full of the most elaborate theories concerning women's issues, but mention feminism and they're horrified: it's unsexy. Young women today assume as their right what their feminist mothers and grandmothers fought for inch by inch." Women notice, remember, and respect men who treat them as equals. Macho behavior is *OUT.*

Psychologist Bernard Zilbergeld interviewed hundreds of women for his book *Men and Sex,* and found that sensitivity was the most sought-after characteristic in a lover:

> I like a partner who can be sensitive to my needs while still being true to his own satisfaction. I like to have my requests listened to and to not be forced into doing things I don't like. In short, I like an equal relationship rather than a one-sided one.

> I like a man who feels free to be vulnerable, to give up his masculine stereotype, who can be gentle and sensitive and passive, as well as aggressive. A man who allows me to do the same. A man who can relinquish

control of the lovemaking and allow it to be a shared experience.

A macho man is fearless, therefore he has no nerves. He is perfectly determined, therefore he has no doubts. He is ruthless in adversity, so it is questionable whether he has a conscience. He is altogether not of flesh and blood. Put him in a Lamborghini, a Ferrari, or a Maserati and he becomes:

Defiant, Courageous, and Fighting Man: DCF Man dreams of thrashing skinheads, punks, and knife-wielding banditos in job lots of a half dozen at a time. He is retarded adolescence. He's also partial to driving at sixty through a thirty-mile-an-hour zone and overtaking three cars at a time on narrow country lanes. Cars, in fact, are the best betrayers of your closet DFC Man, since they're the only means by which he can appear defiant, courageous, and fighting without having to do anything more than moving his foot.

It is a notable fact that when DFC men finally do have their qualities put to the test in an almighty road accident, they either die, go to prison, or become sensible drivers like the rest of us. I have several friends who adhere to the policy that you should never get serious with a man until you see what he's like behind the wheel. (For DFC Man's information, in 1992 in Britain men committed 10,300 indictable driving offenses. Women committed 400.)

"The bigger the hood, the smaller the sex appeal," writes Susannah, who—tall, blond, and rich—is exactly the sort of oo-aah such types hope to lure into their cars. She's quite right to advise men not to waste their wads of cash "on a brand-spanking-new member extension for our sakes. Women are far more likely to be won over by a gentlemanly opening of the passenger door to a beaten-up jalopy that may or may not reach that glorious country hotel for a dirty weekend." Overtly flashy cars hint strongly that the sex will be all thrust and puff.

There are three main ways in which a man, attractive in all other respects, may demote himself in the eyes of a lover. All of them stem from machoness:

1.   He thinks it's unmasculine to show his feelings. She longs for him to be more expressive and less invincible. Here's a true story to illustrate the point. I was reading about a brave soldier called Colonel John Colborne who distinguished himself in the Napoleonic wars. After much fighting, Colborne was shot in the arm by a bullet that also trapped some gold epaulette wire inside him. He endured fifteen months of agony while the doctors made regular, unanesthetized forays into his flesh to try to gouge the items out. Overcome with the trauma of it all, he used occasionally to say to his fellow soldiers, "Give me a glass of wine, I am going to cry." When I read that sentence I fell in love with him immediately, and have remained so to this day.

Nobody wants a man *or* a woman who cries all day long. But showing we are *human* is attractive. That notable weed Tom Hanks is considered a sex bomb because his face and manner show sensitivity. The hulking Liam Neeson too. They emerge as people with concerns, interests, and enthusiasms. A woman immediately feels thoughtful about him as an individual. That's sexy.

2.   He thinks he should be dominant in bed. She, like many of my readers, would like to tie him up, ravish him, and leave him helpless. He would secretly love it if she tied him up, ravished him, and left him helpless, but won't admit it, because the manly way is to lead and instruct. He also thinks getting his penis inside is the most important part of lovemaking. She, as a consequence, finds sex rather dull and predictable, and wishes his penis would take a backseat once in a while.

3.   He thinks it right and "natural" for the male to have superior financial status—and superior intelligence. She finds it very sexy to be able to control the money sometimes, and to get a better grade than he does in night class. He sees this as wanting to emasculate him. She sees it as making life a lot more interesting and can't understand why he can be so touchy; she wasn't touchy when he did better than she did. He thinks of emigrating to America and joining Iron John. She reminds him that also in America is the Denis Thatcher Society, for men married to famous and successful women. "Contrary to what people might think," explains a founding member, "we don't meet to commiserate with each other. We're all very proud of our wives and we think it funny that people believe we're suffering."

Omar Sharif Man falls into this last category. On his side of the bed he had a signed copy of *Omar* ("when he hit Hollywood it was like Valentino reborn") *Sharif: The Eternal Male,* who writes:

> People could get the idea that I have contempt for the weaker sex. The truth is, I worship women . . . but a certain type of woman. The kind who can use both her intelligence and her femininity. A woman mustn't contradict me openly. She must prove to me by some means which I prefer not to know, that I'm wrong and make me change my mind. For instance, by saying to me: "You're right, dear, but don't you think that . . ."
>
> Confronting me head-on, a woman gives me the impression that she's emasculating me.
>
> On the other hand, and I don't think this can be written off as Middle Eastern atavism, I can contradict a woman because I'm a man and because arrogance is in the nature of men.

You've got to hand it to Mr. Sharif, he's frank. The smugness, the gush about respect for femininity, the combination of flattery and patronage, the suggestion that he "understands women"—all the aspects that drive women wild with (nonsexual) frustration.

Women don't want to be worshipped. We don't expect men to "understand" us either, any more than we claim to "understand" men (I certainly don't). Life would be tedious with so much understanding in the air. What women want is a lover to be a friend and partner, as well as a sensitive companion in the bedroom.

How to Keep Her Passion High Once You Get into the Bedroom

Let's assume your cute bottom, slender waist, soulful eyes, and wonderful wittiness have stood you in good stead: the woman of your dreams has agreed to come home with you for the night.

You are still far from home and dry.

Even the sexiest situation can turn suddenly poisonous, if you do the wrong thing as you approach the bed and slip between the sheets. Women's desire is much more delicately balanced than men's: they have been known to run from the room screeching the first excuse that comes to mind because of one small thing that has knocked their passion dead. Oafish behavior is a not infrequent cause of this. Justine, a twenty-eight-year-old courier for a travel firm in Spain, recalls meeting an attractive guy in a bar in the seaside town where she is based, and going home with him. It is not the first such story I have heard.

> We'd already begun to undress when he did something totally unsexy: he farted and didn't bother to cover it up. Didn't look embarrassed, or repentant, nothing. That killed my desire! How could I escape? I hadn't the courage to simply confront him, and I'd just been to the bathroom. Then inspiration came. He turned away and I licked the back of my hand, squashed it against my

eye and smeared my mascara. "Oh God, something in the eye," I blurted. I stumbled out of the room, picked up my coat and was off. What made me especially angry was that he didn't feel he had to bother to be sexy for me. He just assumed I liked him so much. I felt diminished by his attitude, as well as turned off.

Julia had a very different experience:

I'll tell you what he did. We were both students. We'd gotten along well and I was very attracted to him. We went back to his room and were about to get undressed. There was a moth on the wall at about head height. He picked up a soccer ball and bounced it against the wall and killed it. I don't think he was a cruel man really, he thought he was being cool. It made me so sick that I walked out immediately. I couldn't want him after that.

The most common first-night turn-off is undressing badly. Strip like a doofus and all ideas that you are the high-quality lover of her dreams are promptly shattered. Lizzie's man made himself undesirable when "he suddenly started flinging off all his clothes like someone had put itching powder in them. No finesse, no sense of anticipation." Joy remembers her encounter with a lot of laughter:

He was a nice-looking guy, I've thought of him since. But his crime was very simple: he took his pants off too soon. I turned around to find this vision in socks and *shoes,* with short stocky legs and shirttails flapping, neatly folding up his pants!! I mean—yeuk! Luckily his bathroom was connected to the fire escape. I locked myself in and said I had to wash, then crept out down three stories. I lost my best bra but it was worth it. He'd seemed all right at the disco.

In the perfect precoital striptease the externals (coats, jackets, sweaters, etc.) *always* come off first—to be tossed carelessly over the arm of a chair. Don't fuss about hanging it up, doing up the buttons, etc., or she'll think you're (a) persnickety and (b) not sufficiently enthralled. Now the shirt should be loosened *casually,* not as if you simply can't wait to get inside her pants. Too much eagerness is not flattering; it suggests that premature ejaculation will be on the menu. All footwear *must* come off before the pants. Socks, after removal, should be hidden.

At this point even professional male strippers make a basic error. It's essential that you remove your shirt *before* your pants. Men often do it the other way around because that's how they dream of a woman undressing—sexily delicious, prancing about the room in a shirt and bare legs. *Not so men.* Men wearing a shirt and no pants look ridiculous—it's something to do with the way they taper off toward the bottom. So it's shirt off first and then, if you have a nice torso, spend a few minutes strolling about the room apparently searching for something (e.g. where to hide your socks) while she gets to look over the goods.

Now we reach the real danger point: the underwear. Underwear can make or break you in the eyes of a lady, which is why women's magazines are replete with articles about the subject.

I've left a man because of his underwear. We'd been on the floor half clothed and he'd had my panties off and gone down. On the bed when I got his pants down I almost fainted. They were a sort of grubby gray color. There were holes in them.

Even more than holes, women hate underwear that shows too

much. Sexy underwear on a man is discreet, comfortable, not flashy, and not devoted to making his penis the center of attention. Cotton jersey shorts and boxer shorts are the most popular, though the second are reminiscent of gray businessmen in pinstripe suits, and inclined to be decorated with flying elephants, which may or may not go down well. Briefs are boring; they suggest a lack of imagination. Vented briefs are unsexy— "what geeks wear," remarked one knowing underwear spotter. But at the very bottom of the list come thongs, G-strings, and modified shoelaces, which are awful. The British magazine *Woman's Own* panel of experts felt sick at the sight of such flimsy apparel. "Serial killer" wear. "The G-string is horrific. You can tell a lot about a man from the undies he wears and this kind of thing would only be worn by a stripper or a man with a huge ego. If a man I liked wore one of these, I'd grab my bag, make my excuses, and leave." Go for the shorts.

Now take them off.

4

The Woman Unclothed

*E*eeek! Turn out that light!"

The love of your life, caught naked as you sally from the bathroom and flick on the switch, dives behind the curtain and gives Mr. Pudding and his dog from next door an unexpected eyeful. You hold in your mind a blissful flash of curvy flesh, now visible as only a shoulder and arm poking out from the curtain.

"Light! *OFF!*"

"Amanda (Sue, Helen, Lady Jennifer, Mrs. Next-door Neighbor . . .)," you say patiently, "I love to look at you."

Amanda flaps her hand at the switch more vigorously still. Dolefully, you obey.

Women worry about their bodies to a degree that men would think demented. As a concern, it is a hundred times more profound than penis size and baldness put together. Magazines, advertisements, films, bad novels, good novels, television, even lonely hearts columns: all tell us that a sexy woman is slim and flawless. In the words of Sonia, "I feel bombarded by media preoccupations with females and their beauty and sexuality constantly! I try to set my own standards and be happy with myself but it is very hard."

It does not end after you've turned off the light. Amanda

emerges, a substantial phantom, and slithers beneath the comforter just as desired. But when you begin to *feel* what you were not allowed to *see*—her breasts, her hips, her stomach—your hand is skillfully deflected.

One of the most profound bedroom tips a man will ever learn is . . .

MAKE YOUR PARTNER FEEL GOOD ABOUT HER BODY, AND YOUR SEX LIFE WILL IMPROVE BY 100 PERCENT.

Women who feel nervous about their bodies are tense and cautious in bed.

> I'd love to be able to make love with the lights on and mirrors on the ceiling like a sex bomb out of Hollywood. But I ain't got the Hollywood face and figure for it. Bob says I have, but Bob's crazy. The more he says it, the more crazy I know he is.

> I hate my boobs flopping around. My flesh (fat) trembling as two bodies slap together. Having my "love handles" squeezed tight (I'm not fat but could do with toning up—I've always had a good figure and am coming to terms with the beginning signs of aging).

> However much he tells me my body turns him on, all those magazines, advertisements and TV shows convince me that it's ugly because it isn't thin and perfect.

Anxiety about the way we look spoils women's *and* men's sexual pleasure in a dozen ways. Why is she reluctant to go on top? "My breasts are sort of dangling!" Why won't she allow you to penetrate from behind? "I'd *never* let him do that," writes a beautifully proportioned thirty-six-inch-hipped nurse from Norway. "My butt's too big." Why won't she take her nightgown off? "I'm overweight from just having a baby and worried that I may not feel the same to him." Dress up in sexy underwear? "I would feel like such an idiot. I'm no Claudia Schiffer." Do it outside in a field of wildflowers? "Too thin, breasts aren't big enough, etc." Do it under the stars, by the glow of the moon? "I'm fat." (She's five foot nine and weighs 134 pounds—she's underweight.) When a woman mysteriously won't participate in something sexual with her partner, odds are it's because she thinks it makes her look unattractive. Women who disapprove of sexual practices for other reasons usually say so: "No, I'm not pretending to be Batwoman and dangling from the stairwell, it's perverted." But nobody wants to draw attention to the fact that they feel fat and bulgy.

I know the problems intimately. I researched the subject in detail for my book *Fabulous Figures: Or How to Be Utterly Uniquely Gorgeous,* in which I discuss women's self-critical attitudes to their own figures, dieting, beauty, and health. The fact is, nearly all women nowadays feel bad about some part of their body, if not all of it. Ninety-five percent of *How to Have an Orgasm* readers cited figure worries at the top of their list of sexual hang-ups. Yet such anxieties usually bear little or no relation to what the woman actually looks like. Therefore, you *can* help.

Flab always comes at the top of the list of concerns. Women consistently overrate how stout they are, and find it hard to believe what their friends and family tell them. Even women with perfect bodies see themselves as "untoned," "fat," "wobbly," and "revolting." They send me photos of themselves—wonderfully attractive faces and figures that any man would be proud to entertain, and on the back they write: "Me. My 'before' picture. Aren't I disgusting? Send you another when I'm perfect."

The pressure nowadays is greater than ever before. It's not simply that women are supposed to "be attractive" in general. Beauty gurus focus on every single detail of our bodies: we must have slim legs, flawless skin, flat tummies (bad luck if you've got three lovely children), a suntan without the peeling nose, long red talons, feet that look as if they've never seen a shoe, elbows with no dry flaky bits on them, and *of course* no cellulite (if you don't know what cellulite is I'm *certainly* not going to tell you). Recently to all that has been added just-the-right-amount-of-muscle-i.e.-about-as-much-as-Madonna-has. It's utterly exhausting.

Men are far more tolerant of women's variousness than women are. Most wouldn't even notice, let alone care, whether their lover's waist is twenty-six inches or twenty-eight; but the difference will cause a woman months of anguish. Being "too fat" is women's number one physical concern. In the words of Ogden Nash:

> Some ladies smoke too much and
> Some ladies drink too much and
> Some ladies pray too much
> But all ladies think that they weigh too much.

So they diet constantly. And dieting makes the anxiety worse.

"But," you might protest, "if a woman worries about being too fat, then surely the best thing she can do is diet and she'll become thin and happy."

Alas, this is known as the Wrong Approach.

Dieting Makes Things Worse

Suggest that a woman diets—imply, thereby, that she is fat and ungainly—and you might as well buy yourself a one-way ticket to a monastery. Intimacy, affection, and raunchy romps with the light on will all diminish in direct proportion to your enthusiasm for the idea. Dieting—i.e., the severe restriction of calories needed to produce discernible weight loss in a short period of time—reduces sex drive and causes divorces. From a happy, re-laxed woman she becomes a nervy, bad-tempered, self-critical, calorie-pinching dieter. And don't think she's going to be the only one who has to eat the filthy diet food—it'll be lowfat yo-gurt and taste-free "health" bars all around.

If your lover succeeds in dieting her way to a weight she's happy with, a rare but not impossible occurrence, she'll be there as on a precipice. For a while she'll be wild and free. She'll take to wandering about the house admiring herself in every scrap of mirror in sight. Out will come wardrobes of col-orful clothes that you never knew she possessed. Frilly lingerie will be reintroduced. Give her a bottle of wine, and she'll be only too happy to frolic nude at the bottom of the bed, pre-tending she's a belly dancer in your harem.

This state of affairs will last about a month.

Then the weight will come back. It always does. Take heed of Ms. M. H.: "I've probably gained and lost 1,000 pounds in my life."

No, let me be precise about this. In 95–98 percent of cases of dieting, the weight lost returns, usually within months, and often *with interest*. All those lovely clothes will miraculously vanish again, the lacy panties will once more be squashed at the back of the sensible underwear drawer, and half a crate of wine won't secure any extravagances at all, save a blackout. To the familiar worries about love handles and wobbly bottoms will be added a sense of failure and self-distaste.

Diets are passion killers.

The Correct Approach to making a woman feel good about her body is to take exactly the opposite tactic. Counterintuitive though this might seem at first, it is nevertheless the way for-ward. Discourage dieting. Hold ritualistic burnings of the latest diet fad books. Make sure the car breaks down every time she's due at her weight loss club meeting. No degree of sabotage should be left untried.

Here's a bit more ammunition for the battle against diet disease. Consider them the articles of war, to be read out each night before bed, so that she may mull over them in the weakened hours of her sleep.

1. Dieting makes her fat. The paradoxical postulate is the strongest arrow in a man's quiver. Point out that after a diet much of the weight that returns is fat, even if most of what departed was muscle. This is because the body is making a quick attempt to build up stores of energy before she decides to do such a stupid thing again, and fat accumulation is the easiest way to do it. Then harp on about the 95–98 percent failure rate (or the 2–5 percent success rate; for the greatest impression I suggest alternating the two). This has been firmly established by dozens of controlled experiments around the world. The more dramatic the diet, the worse the damage. Those "Lose 10 lb in 10 days" boasts should be avoided like the plague.

Diets also cause panic reactions. Where once she was quite happy to eat three cookies with her coffee, on a diet she will nobly eat *no* cookies; after five hours of a rumbling stomach and tantalizing dreams of dancing chocolate treats, her willpower will suddenly snap. She'll rush to the kitchen and wolf the whole package.

2. Dieting is bad for her. Rattle out the following: the height-weight charts are a load of garbage first invented by insurance companies to massage their profits; they are not scientifically sound and are widely condemned by specialists. As well as low sex drive, dieting can cause cancer, cardiovascular disease, osteoporosis, aging (that's a good one to dwell on), gallstones, mental illness, and suicide. The largest detailed health study ever conducted—on 1.8 million people in 1984 in Norway—concluded that women who weigh twice as much as the usual weight chart recommendation live longer than those goody-goodies in the so-called ideal range.

Weight of woman	Chance of living to sixty-five
110 lb	73.0 percent
122 lb	82.4 percent
224 lb plus	84.4 percent
280 lb plus	75.7 percent

Dieting also causes infertility. Scientists have known for a long time that women who are too thin lose the ability to have children. Recently, it's been found that ordinary-weight women who diet too much also lose their fertility. The body decides it can't trust this person to be a mother.

None of this is guaranteed to stick, but one must not give up hope. If you cure her of diet disease, you will be three-

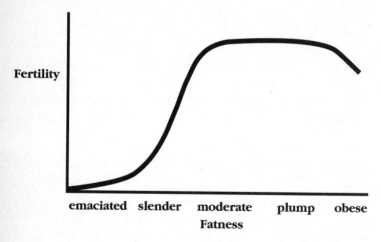

Graph to show the relationship between fertility and fatness. Important for the explanation of why plumpness was so universally admired before the latter half of this century. Useful for showing to girlfriends and hopeful moms whose idea of a body is two hipbones and a washboard of ribs. (Taken from J. L. Anderson et al., "Was the Duchess of Windsor Right?" in *Ethology and Sociobiology* 13, 1992.)

quarters of the way toward making her feel happy about her body and wild in bed. It is easier to change attitudes about your body than it is to lose weight successfully. When women stop feeling under pressure to diet they often find (as I did) that a more relaxed attitude to food results in weight loss without trying.

Nevertheless, I am by no means against weight loss if it *really* will improve a person's life. There are occasions when your partner feels justifiably unhappy as she is, or when her size is inconvenient. If she's dead set on it, then your job is to encourage her to lose the weight gradually and sensibly. Instead of a crash diet (which will fail), insist that she change her eating habits gently. Give her every support, i.e., don't tuck into meatloaf, with a hot fudge sundae and whipped cream for dessert, whenever she tries to eat a salad and poached fish. Join in. Even if you're already slim, it's important to remember that *thinness is not the same as good health*. What you eat is just as important as what shape you are.

Other Tactics for Making a Woman Happy about Her Body

I have already mentioned that women who are convinced that they are fat pay little heed to what other people say. As her lover you are in the best position to make an impression, but even here additional tactics are extremely important and to be adopted at all times.

1. Don't be pushy: Don't insist that she expose herself naked in bright light, just because you know she's silly to be so modest. This does not mean you are doomed to perpetual darkness. Overcome her aversion gradually. Replace the 500-watt halogen bulb that beams down on her buttocks with a very, very low light and work upward. Don't demand to make love with her in red lace underwear. *Woman's Own* magazine knew its market when it ran a feature entitled "He Wants Me Vampy . . . I Want to Hide My Bulges." Elaborate sex-crazed lingerie may look good on a model, but many women feel silly and overexposed wearing it themselves, and garters can be fiendishly uncomfortable. Confidence has to be built up in stages. There are many more concealing sexy garments available (begin looking in Victoria's Secret). A man's long shirt looks just as alluring on an otherwise naked woman.

Making love partially or fully clothed is another good way of getting around a woman's nervousness about overexposure. Writes auburn-haired, 39-27-36 Carolyn:

> I never thought I'd have sex outside before I met my last boyfriend, but now we do it all the time. We've "baptized" all the woods and fields in the area, and always with my clothes on. He pushes my panties away and enters. I had him on a plane from California when I sat on his lap. Who said you need nudity?

2.   Flattery: Men *never* get this right. It's such a simple thing, so easy to do, yet you're all terrible at it. Use nice straightforward sincerity. The Omar Sharif Man who purrs sugary compliments into a woman's ear is embarrassing: "Dah-leeng, I lurva your eyes, they are like the sea of life, dragging me under" (cringe).

People love to be told they're marvelous. *Tell* her you enjoy her body. Tell her *regularly*. As in: "I love you," "You're so sexy," "Mmmmmmm," "Aaaaaaaaah," etc. Begin now. Praise flows even more smoothly and sincerely after you've wet your whistle. Also flatter her indirectly, by long concentration on those particular parts that entice you, kissing, stroking, and displaying an unwillingness to tear yourself away. I guarantee such behavior will pay dividends: good sex is 50 percent confidence. If you're of an orderly frame of mind, keep a diary. Note down the number of times she praises you, and match or better it. Men expect to be flattered and encouraged, so you'll be surprised how much work you have to do to keep up with her.

One of the classic problems between the sexes is that the man assumes the woman knows he likes her and thinks she's lovely. This should never be relied upon, not least because women always exaggerate their own bad features. She might have been certain of your affection once, but people's feelings change and a ten-year-old compliment just won't do. She *doesn't* know unless you tell her frequently. In a recent edition of *Options* magazine several couples were asked to keep secret records of their sex lives:

Karen: I asked Daniel if he thought I was less attractive now. He looked me up and down and said he'd still have sex with me, which didn't really answer the question.

Daniel: She seems to think I don't desire her anymore. But if I didn't find her so sexy, I wouldn't constantly be trying to get her into bed. I like Karen a lot and would like to make love more.

I could brain this man. Why on earth couldn't he have spoken frankly to his wife instead of to his diary?!! Lack of flattery is a significant factor in driving people to adultery. Women (and men) frequently have affairs simply to boost their self-esteem. It is very nice to find a bit on the side who'll say silly things about you again.

By the same token the opposite of flattery—criticism—is never profitable. Criticism can be indirect and may not be intended as criticism at all. It is often distilled from comments you've made about other people, and can undo in an instant all the good work you've put in:

I have fantastic legs and a beautiful aristocratic face. I like my neck and hair and I'm all right with my breasts. My husband repeatedly tells me I am beautiful and always has a creative compliment on hand . . . But I feel fat (five foot two, 130–135 lb). I know I'm passable with clothes on but I'm not getting naked for anyone. Ick. I worry my husband will feel my tummy during sex. I know he is very picky about what is pretty or too fat by the critical way he speaks of other women and even himself (he was a fat kid).

I usually feel a little self-conscious during sex unless it is very dark. I don't want my boyfriend to see my cellulite. I am fairly slim but I do have cellulite on my thighs and butt. He is very observant and critical of people that are overweight or flabby. I fear that if he sees my flab, he will no longer be attracted to me . . .

That husband and boyfriend are their own worst enemies. Every time a man criticizes another person's body, his partner transfers the criticism to herself. He probably doesn't even realize it.

3. Don't Ogle: Ogling other women is a turn-off. Men go wild with jealousy if a girlfriend does it, but think it perfectly right and natural to indulge in themselves. Do as you would be done by. The more you ogle women, the less your partner relaxes in bed and the worse everything becomes.

Ogling includes gawking at models in the *Sports Illustrated* swimsuit issue, pinning up pictures of Sharon Stone next to the razor mirror, and remarking that you'd give your left arm to spend an hour with Michelle Pfeiffer. It's no good saying that these are merely innocent comments about another woman's attractiveness that in no way reflect a criticism of your girlfriend—it won't wash. Ogling is criticism whether you intend it that way or not. It simply adds to the pressure she feels from everywhere else, demanding that a proper woman should lose weight, get a face-lift, and change bodies with the latest streak of catwalk spaghetti.

> Women notice who men are looking at. I always notice when he does it. It seizes me up, and if he's been staring at a thinner or more attractive woman sex is always worse that night. It would make him nervous if I did the same back, but I don't.

> Men who gawk at other women when you're out with them are terrible for me. They're unsexy and you always feel like you're being compared to the glossy picture or every short skirt in the street. That feeling persists. In bed, you think: "Is he thinking my legs aren't as long as the woman we met in the supermarket? Better cover them up." It always rebounds on the men in the end.

There is only one circumstance in which ogling can be used to good effect. If you have a roving eye, then train it to rove this way . . .

4. Positive Ogling is a refined form of flattery and requires skill. Basically, the idea is that you make a point of ogling those women who have an ample portion of whatever it is your girlfriend criticizes most about herself, e.g., big hips, large breasts (or, conversely, boyishness), curvy thighs, strong nose, etc. It's not difficult to do. I'm frequently admiring ultra-skinny men, which usually results in my boyfriend feeling extra cheerful, not bothering with his exercises for the next five days, and jumping into bed with me instead. "I make one exception to the roving eye man," says Loretta. "If he looks at people like me. I'm black and statuesque. What's it going to do to me if he stares at thin whiteys? But if he flatters me by looking at other big black women, that's okay."

All other ogling, if you must do it, should be confined to when your partner's not with you. But remember, women who are ogled rarely find it flattering. If I notice a man sneaking discreet looks at me, that's sexy. Outright oglers are crude and intrusive. Ogling is the visual equivalent of scratching your groin.

5

Fiddling

License my roving hands, and let them go
Before, behind, between, above, below.
—JOHN DONNE

*F*oreplay strikes terror into brave men's hearts. It is (supposedly) the fussy, feminine part of sex that has to go on forever and ever before the manly rutting can begin; and if it goes wrong then one's reputation as a sensitive lover goes out the window forever.

I find the very word a turn-off, which is why I've titled this chapter Fiddling. "Foreplay" reeks of humorless sex therapy, manages to be both goody-goody and seedy, and brings to mind fore*skin,* not the most attractive feature of male anatomy. Most important of all, "foreplay" is a misnomer: it suggests that intercourse is the "point" of sex and this is just a little warm-up. "Fiddling" is much more to the point: simply the erotic things women and men do to each other *apart* from penetration. It can happen before, during, after, or in place of intercourse. Fiddling is as sexy as your skill and imagination can make it, and even the most unromantic societies indulge in it. The Sirionos of South America don't believe in love, but "a certain amount of affection does exist between the sexes," remarks a learned anthropologist. "This is clearly reflected in the behavior that takes place around the hammock . . . scratching and pinching each other on the neck and chest, poking fingers in each other's eyes . . ."

Why Do Women Want Fiddling?

The practical answer is that it hots us up and slows you down. As soon as the penis is inside a woman, the threat of it ejaculating and putting a premature end to the business increases dramatically. With a bit of care, fiddling allows the man to keep erect and give the woman immense pleasure while staving off his orgasm. Presto! Three-minute man is turned into the equivalent of a sexual marathon runner.

Fiddling is also the languor before the storm. It is the period in which the partners are together as patient, careful lovers and a woman gets to use all her senses erotically. Intercourse, however passionate, has a tendency to be impersonal: sensation concentrated around the hips, orgasm on the near horizon. During fiddling, the sensations are diffuse, gentle, and intimate. This is a theme that crops up again and again.

> Foreplay [i.e., fiddling] is emotion and intercourse is physical. Foreplay is for lovers and intercourse (on its own) is for strangers.

> It's my way of showing I care about Peter, every bit of him, savoring him inch by inch, his smell, his feel, his very essence. There's no way I want that kind of intimacy with any ole guy however big his dick.

> If I have a lot of sex play with a man it's because I want to explore him all over and want to be explored myself. I like to play with all those parts that get overlooked

during intercourse. It's very full. Very calm (or explosive!) and fulfilling.

For those who have difficulty reaching orgasm, fiddling is particularly relaxing and delicious:

> This is my time, all for me. I don't have to concentrate about getting my satisfaction or worrying that he's going to come too soon, yet.

> Like all women I love sensual men. A man who kisses my neck, my breasts, who runs his hands over my whole body is a man who will make love beautifully. A crude man, even if he went on humping all night, wouldn't make me pop.

Fiddling doesn't have to be concentrated or continuous, and can be interrupted by coffee breaks if desired, but it should be unhurried. The point is not merely to push each other to the peak of arousal, but to ensure that every part of the body becomes involved in the experience. Good sex "grows out" of the circumstances: it is not something unconnected with other activities. Fiddling should be gradual. It should not focus on getting to the fucking stage as quickly as possible:

> I always say: "Foreplay begins the moment you meet a sexy man." It's all foreplay. Intimate touching is an extension of intimate conversation which is an extension of ordinary comments about the weather uttered with knowing, anticipatory glances at each other.

> I hate the word foreplay because it means that it's not the real thing. It *is* the real thing. You can come during foreplay, can't you? Coming's the real thing, isn't it? In an ideal world, intercourse would be nothing special. There's oral, manual, between the breasts, between the

thighs, mutual masturbation. Foreplay is a bit of all of these, working up to orgasm.

Foreplay is flirting with your clothes off.

Women's Most Erogenous Zone

> Two lovers sat in a café. He asked her if she had any special erogenous zones. Perplexed, she frowned a little as she carefully reviewed all the places where she liked to be touched. Then she smiled and said, "Skin— anywhere on my skin."
>
> —BEATRICE FAUST, *WOMEN, SEX AND*
> *PORNOGRAPHY*

Women want to be touched. Not by men on the subway during the rush hour, or by fumblers at parties crowding around the drinks table, pretending to be filling up their wineglass, but by the men we choose to go to bed with. More than any specific thing, women like the feeling of a man's hand moving gently, playing with our hair, stroking our arms and backs, down between our breasts . . . around our waist . . . his kisses down the whole length of our thighs . . . (and so on). One of the main reasons bisexual women are more likely to climax with another woman than with a man is because not enough male lovers understand this fact.

We are the tactile sex: women's skin is thinner and more sensitive than men's, which may be due to the female sex hormone estrogen. After menopause (when estrogen levels drop), women lose some of their skin sensitivity; they regain it if they go on hormone replacement therapy (HRT). Jan Morris, the travel writer who was born male and had a sex-change operation, describes her experiences after taking female hormones for several years, when body hair, "leathery skin," and hard muscle protrusions all vanished:

> . . . but there went with them something less tangible too, which I know now to be something specifically masculine—a kind of unseen layer of accumulated resilience, which provides a shield for the male species, but at the same time deadens the sensations of the body . . . This suggestion, for it is really hardly more, was now stripped from me, and I felt at the same time physically freer and more vulnerable. I had no armour.

Some women are so sensitive to touch that they have climaxed simply by having their teeth, eyebrows, or hair played with! "I have never had an orgasm during intercourse, though I have had what I believe to be one standing up having my neck stroked," writes one woman. I personally think feet are the most sensuous part of the body.

Touch, in all its forms, is incredibly important to women in a sexual relationship. Too little kissing, for example, is one of the most common complaints women make about their sex lives. Many consider the kiss to be the most intimate of all acts, so much so that prostitutes pride themselves on not kissing clients, even when they will do anything else. (The Thonga of Mozambique view kissing in a quite different light: "Look at them," they said when they first saw two Westerners engaged in this curious activity, "they eat each other's saliva and dirt.") "I like to be kissed *all* over by my boyfriend," says Laura. "Gently, languidly, from head to foot." All-over touching and kissing is never merely sexual (as straightforward genital contact is): it is a display of emotional closeness. It leads to blissful relationships as well as blissful sex.

All women do not like to be treated in the same way, however, so proceed with care. Some women hate having their breasts twiddled with. Others go wild about particular places . . . inner surfaces of the thighs, tongue, abdomen, center of the lower back, behind the knees, soles of feet, palms and fingertips.

A quick peck on the lips as we're coming up the stairs to the apartment, snatched on the landing. Sometimes he'll press me against the wall and demand more. We open a bottle of wine and drink it as he undresses me. I like to feel myself completely naked and vulnerable while he's still dressed. He is very gentle. He covers every inch of me in kisses and licks—*every* inch.

Foreplay must be slow and it must not be genitally centered. It should be savored. It should often be instead of intercourse. The best time ever for me was when Bob and me just kept going. I came and we kept going, then he came and afterwards kept stroking me. We had a meal. Afterwards we kept going. There was no goal. We just eventually fell asleep in each other's arms.

I like it best when he starts kissing my neck and back, then gradually works down to my genitals and makes me climax like that. But not the same way each time, please! That would be boring.

It's nice to have a massage lying on my front then when I feel totally relaxed he enters me from behind. Once I fell asleep because he was giving me such a good massage and woke to find him inside me in the last stages of pleasure! Otherwise I think foreplay should be like a game and never too serious.

He starts saying what he's going to do to me when we're out with friends. Whispers in my ear: "I'm going to put my mouth between your legs" or "I'm going to fuck you until you beg me to stop." I find that a real turn-on. When we get home we undress each other, very affectionate. No rushing. He sucks my breasts. Kisses me under the chin, prods my feet. It can go on for an hour or five minutes, depending on how we feel and whether I'm desperate to be penetrated or not. We've spent the whole evening doing sexual things and other things as well, and that's very nice.

Women also get immense pleasure from doing the touching, so be patient when she spends a languid half hour stroking you all over. It's not time "wasted," as one most *un*sensuous man remarked. It's adding hugely to her sexual arousal and it will also add to yours. I quote here a revealing letter I received from a reader:

I presently work as a massage therapist and this has opened my eyes and been a bigger education than anything. Ninety-nine percent of the men want a hand release. For the last six months I was very definite about not doing it—most accepted it, some got upset about it. It seems to me that men come for a massage not because they've got sore muscles but because it's a way they can get the touching they want (and maybe don't want to admit they want)—even if they're in a relationship. And sometimes my client might have had his wife die suddenly and so the touching is truly therapeutic.

After six months of holding out and being righteous I started relaxing a bit and began thinking—well, it's just another part of the body. But for me it's important that I feel good about the person so I do tell some men that I don't do that. Mostly I have really nice clients. A couple of them I've got to be friends with and these are the ones where I've got into playing with them a little— tying them up and teasing them—but I don't make love with them. It's with these ones that we've talked about fantasies and what we like and don't like and it's helped me to talk with people who have no fear of saying they like something or that something turns them on. I feel that I'm getting more and more in touch with my sexuality and especially doing massage for the last year. I get turned on by some of my clients and I get turned on when some of them come. It's been interesting to feel my body responding—and I guess the bit that men wouldn't understand is that I don't feel frustrated if I don't have an orgasm then or that day.

Breasts

An important feature in the fiddling process.

Bosoms, boobs, knockers, tits, melons, lemons, milkshakes, lungs, lulus, bazooms, cat and kitties, Tale of Two Cities, thousand pities . . . call them what you will, the universal truism about Those Two Things That Stick Out is: those of us who have plenty wish for less, and those who have little long for more. Women go through agonies about their figures, and bosoms are high on the list of anxiety inducers. For example, do they pass the Pencil-Test? (Work that one out for yourself.) Are they pointed/rounded/high/together/smooth/identical enough?

On a diet, boobs are the first things to suffer, and bosom pride has saved many a woman from the indignity of starving herself. Conversely, there is no way to increase their size or improve their tone naturally. Exercising only strengthens the muscles underneath, it does nothing for the things themselves. "Bust-enhancing" creams and potions used to be advertised a lot in the 1950s and 1960s, but they merely temporarily inflame the skin and make it appear puffed up (as Andy, in chapter 6, painfully discovered). Without surgery, a woman is stuck with the bosoms God gave her. As they are closely tied up with our self-esteem, another golden rule for the good lover is

---

BE NICE TO YOUR PARTNER'S BOSOMS.

Praise them lavishly. Make a virtue of their distinctive features. And *never, never* encourage her to have breast implants. It's a painful and risky business, absolutely her decision and not yours. Cindy Jackson, who in her pursuit of wanting to look like a Barbie doll has had over twenty operations and has spoken openly about her cosmetic surgery, describes how she

> had a one-and-a-half-inch incision made underneath each breast. The surgeon inserted his hands and made a pocket. The silicone implant was placed behind the muscle on the wall of my chest. It was then sewn up, leaving a tiny scar. It was very painful. After the operation I felt sick and my breasts felt hot and swollen— they looked like missiles. I could hardly move for days.
>
> The results disappointed me . . . Three months later the left breast became hard and painful. Scar tissue was forming around the implant. Surgeons broke it free by twisting it—it was agony. Half of the implant then slipped behind the muscle, making my breasts un-even . . .

Implants can leak; they can mask early cancer signs; they can cause an enormous range of ghastly problems. A woman having the operation may lose sensation in her breasts, and there is a one in five chance that her nipples will become necrotic and drop off.

Between 10 and 20 percent of women can have an orgasm by breast stimulation alone (usually stroking, kissing, and sucking). It is not uncommon for women to have orgasms while breast-feeding (some have even climaxed during childbirth), though our social mores prevent us from dwelling on the fact.

There is nothing disgusting or unnatural about this: breast-feeding, birth, and sexual arousal each involve the same hormonal and neurological pathways. However, approach bosoms with care: excessive squeezing, knocking, and pounding *hurt*.

About 40 percent of women don't enjoy having their breasts touched, and some of those are particularly squeamish about their nipples. This sensitivity sometimes depends on which position the woman's breasts are in—they tend to be more sensitive when she is lying flat than when standing up. If you feel nervous about your talents in the nipple-fondling department, *The Sensuous Man,* by "M," has the perfect answer: practice on a grape.

> Place a small grape in your mouth. Keeping it between your teeth and your tongue, rotate it with your tongue. Be extremely careful not to break the skin of the grape. Roll it from side to side in your mouth and knead it with your lips. When you are able to manipulate the grape in this fashion without rupturing the skin, then you are applying approximately the correct amount of pressure necessary to stimulate and excite her nipples without causing any pain to these very sensitive erogenous zones. If you are able to bring the grape to orgasm so much the better.

A lot of nonsense is written about "erect nipples" signifying sexual desire. Sometimes they do, sometimes they don't. It is perfectly possible for women to be highly aroused, even to have an orgasm, and have no sign of erect nipples. Conversely, nipples that are erect may signify nothing more than that the bedroom needs to be warmer. Being cold does wonders for bosoms generally—it firms and tightens them, which is one reason why shots of wet models in the sea are so popular. Men who enjoy stimulating their penis between a woman's breasts may find it works best in a cool place.

Some conversation-stopping facts about boobs: they evolved from sweat glands, so that milk, like vaginal lubrication, is really just a form of modified sweat. One unsettled question is why the human female is the only primate to have such big 'uns. It's not for reproductive purposes, since flat-chested women are just as capable of producing milk. Could it be for sexual ones? Chest size has no relation to chest sensitivity, but several imaginative scientists have proposed that bosoms are designed to mimic buttocks and so incite men approaching from the front to hurry around back and whip their willies out. This, they say, is a relic of the poor-postured days of humanity, when sex from the rear was the only feasible position. Various apes and monkeys are cited to support the thesis, because they have lurid red markings on their chests, which look very like their reproductive organs at the rear. It's not awfully convincing.

Pigs have between fourteen and eighteen breasts. The coypu has them on her back. The average human breast weighs 7 oz, except after childbirth when it goes up to a whopping 17 oz; however, almost all women have one breast bigger than the other. Nipples are also curious. They can, theoretically, grow anywhere along two lines in the body known as "milk lines," which extend in a gentle curve from the armpits down to the groin. Most people have just two, but about one in twenty men have a third, and there are records of women having up to eight pairs of functioning breasts.

Why do men have nipples? Because women do. Nipples in both sexes develop from the same structure in the sexless embryo. In a man they are simply a relic of this early time and serve no purpose. According to one writer, different types of men have different nipple preferences.

High-class intellectuals and complex sensualists usually want women with small pink nipples; strong male animals prefer brown nipples, while men who have once been orphan children or are sorrowing widowers, liked to rest in the shadow of large, red nipples. The real stags—those who don't care what kind of woman they embrace—have, of course, no preference.

—GEORGE FALUDI, *MY HAPPY DAYS IN HELL*

A Woman's Lower Regions

Fiddling, like any other weighty matter, progresses earthward. After kissing and breasts (although, of course, the good lover must not make it appear so systematic) come the highly sensitive and complex lower regions.

Although men and women look like they're poles apart in terms of sexual characteristics, there are many physical comparisons that can be made because both male and female sex organs originate from the same embryonic blob. The ovaries, for example, are the female counterpart of the testes, which is why a huge penis, or a deep pelvic thrust during intercourse that knocks against the ovaries, is so painful to a woman: it feels to her as a man feels when he's been kicked in the balls. Other counterparts are the scrotum and the major lips of the vulva; and the foreskin and the clitoral hood. These are shown in the stylized diagram opposite.

The drawing on the left is of the vulva, the umbrella name for all the external female sex organs. The vulva extends from the mons veneris, or mount Venus, down to the perineum, which is the part between the vaginal entrance and the anus, about halfway between a woman's legs. For those of you with a particularly innocent past and no TV, I should warn you that the real article is covered in hair. The Victorian art historian John Ruskin, who learned his female anatomy from statues, was so horrified on his wedding night to discover that his wife had not the smooth baldness of marble that he promptly became impotent.

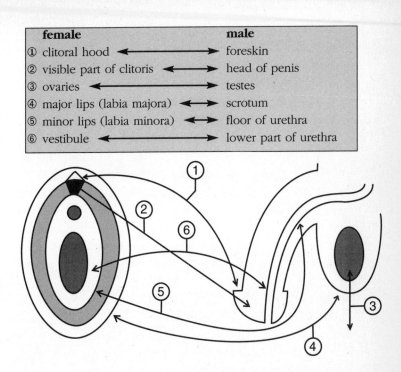

female	male
① clitoral hood ←————→	foreskin
② visible part of clitoris ←——→	head of penis
③ ovaries ←————→	testes
④ major lips (labia majora) ←→	scrotum
⑤ minor lips (labia minora) ←→	floor of urethra
⑥ vestibule ←————→	lower part of urethra

Diagram showing the counterparts in women's and men's sexual organs.

The mons veneris and the labia majora have a large number of nerve endings and are therefore very responsive to erotic stimulation. The labia minora also has lots of nerves, but you have to be a little more cautious with how you play around here. Some women find that, unless aroused already, direct contact is painful rather than pleasurable. (The vagina will be discussed in chapter 7, "Penetration.")

The clitoris is the female counterpart of the penis. The bulk of the clitoral system is actually inside a woman's body and just like the penis, it swells during sexual arousal. "In short," writes Shere Hite, "the only real difference between men's and women's erections is that men's are on the outside of their bodies, while women's are on the inside." The visible clitoris, about an inch long, is like the tip of a woman's "penis." What's more, it contains roughly the same number of nerves as a man has in his organ, in a much, much smaller volume, which is why badly performed manual sex is such agony for a woman.

The only human organ devoted entirely to erotic pleasure, the clitoris was "discovered" in 1593 by Realdus Columbus, exactly one century after his namesake Christopher discovered America. How was it, marveled Realdus, "so many noted anatomists overlooked so pretty and useful a thing?" Yet only in the last forty years has science "confirmed" what all masturbating women since 25,000 B.C. have known, namely, that for the vast majority of women, stimulation of the clitoris is essential for orgasm.

The clitoris is extremely difficult to find and many women don't know where theirs is. Whenever I am feeling really pissed off with the male sex and thinking of turning lesbian, one thing stops me: the prospect of the dreaded search for *someone else's* clitoris. Back to heterosex forthwith! It's hardly surprising, therefore, that men have difficulty. Think you know the spot? Ha! This is no time to get smug. During sexual arousal it swells and increases in length and diameter, particularly at the tip, and then, just before climax . . . it vanishes. This odd behavior can be disconcerting:

> "Not there . . . up a little . . . that's the spot . . . now easy . . . no, lower. Lower! O! O!" She made some joy sounds, then cursed. "I don't know what's wrong! You hit the spot every night and morning last week! Now you can't seem to find it at all!"
>
> "But maybe it's just not there any more."
>
> "No, it is! It is! You just don't know where to try."
>
> "But I am trying. I did try. The spot's moved. Here,

let me try again. My jowls are throbbing. Stell—Stradella.
I can't find it. I can't!"

"No, it hasn't moved! It hasn't. It's still there! You
don't know where to look. Keep trying. Keep looking."
—JAMES SHERWOOD, *STRADELLA*

Remember, remember: the clitoris is *not* a magic button.
Many men believe it is and press it energetically: they are duly
rewarded with the woman writhing and moaning . . . in agony.
In my younger days when I was too polite to speak up I endured this torture many times. It's particularly bad from so-
called "sexperts." Shy, inexperienced fellows tend to proceed
with more caution. In some women the clitoris is so sensitive
that direct touching is extremely painful; in others, direct and
vigorous manipulation is pleasurable, even necessary for orgasm, but can leave them feeling sore for several days afterward. Men, accustomed to applying vigorous pleasure to their
clitoral counterpart the penis, understandably find it hard to appreciate just how different the two things actually are.

Performing Manual Sex on a Woman

The most important thing to remember for manual sex is what
you have just read about the clitoris: it is *highly sensitive* down
there. Every woman's nightmare is the man who fumbles
around between her legs, latches onto that protruding bit, and
then rubs away like a French polisher. Women who like it
rough will usually say so, so unless she urges you to press
harder, keep it soft. One woman found she had most success
when her husband used his flaccid penis against her (there are
many uses for a limp penis).

The trick with manual sex is to begin with general stimulation, since virtually all pressure that is more or less in the right
area (i.e., between the legs or just above) will move the vagi-

nal lips, which are attached to the clitoris hood, which will, in turn, stimulate the clitoris beneath. Michelle, a doctor who wrote me an eleven-page letter, including a photograph of herself bungee-jumping in New Zealand, offers the following sensible words of advice:

> In my experience the best manual sex with a guy you don't know comes when you've still got your panties on. If the guy isn't quite sure what he's doing the panties even out his mistakes. He can't get too focused, and he usually ends up just rubbing the general area, which is grand, because that's all I want. That's all I need. It's also good like this if you want to keep the sex kind of aloof, like at a disco or a dinner party or something. Just Paul's hand teasing me through my underwear is great!

When the woman is more aroused, has got you doing it how she likes, and wants more focused attention, she can either take her underclothes off or slip your hand beneath her panties.

Sans underclothes, again continue with indirect pressure, and then let your partner vary the intensity and place as she indicates. If you sit between a woman's legs and imagine the vulva as a clock, with twelve o'clock (the clitoris) uppermost, you'll find that most women are particularly sensitive to stimulation at the four o'clock and eight o'clock positions. At these two points, there are nerve bundles in the lips on both sides of the vagina. The G-spot is about two inches inside the vagina, at the twelve o'clock position, but remember that most women don't find it at all special. It is not just that different women are differently sensitive, but also that numerous factors can make any individual woman's sensitivity change considerably from one night to the next. Time of the month, various complaints such as yeast infection or cystitis, too much sex the evening before—these factors can turn what was once a pleasurable experience into a very painful one. Go slow. Test her responses:

> Just massage over the area, back and forth, up and down, with a bit more pressure on the fingertips. Keep it moving and keep the pussy closed, like the whole place was like a pair of flesh panties instead of cotton ones. When I get close, I want it harder and near the vagina itself I find, but that's just me. I'd prefer it if his penis goes in when I come too, because it gives me something to grip on to and that makes it pleasurable.

Another common mistake made during manual sex is to assume that the woman immediately wants to be penetrated: in goes the finger and lashes about a bit until she collapses in a groan of irritation or forces you to move on to more promising things. The repellent phrase "finger-fucking" refers to this schoolboy sport, and it is always a disaster. "When I was a teenager," remembers Sidonie, from Paris, "I thought there was something wrong with me. Here the fellow was wiggling his forefinger around inside me like a baby eel and all I wanted to do was laugh and hit him on the head. I felt I had vaginal worms or something." Penetration with a finger can be sexy, but not alone.

> I remember one: it was wonderful, my lover used his finger and stroked my clitoris (told me that's what it was, until then I thought it was where I peed from!!!) then plunged it (finger) into my pussy (which was very aroused—we'd just had sex and I hadn't come). I remember thinking afterwards that my pelvic area was in control when suddenly it automatically bucked—no conscious message came from my head, then pow! Orgasm.

If you find you cannot manage to arouse your partner by manual sex, don't worry. First, it is not universally popular. Second, *it is extremely difficult to do exactly right*. Few men can be as skilled in this department as the woman is with herself. (Oral sex is a different matter!)

> I love to do manual sex to my partner because I really enjoy looking at his penis . . . but I have to accept that he cannot arouse me to the same level I can myself (I would have to give him incredibly detailed instructions to the exact millimeter!). He knows this too but enjoys "exploring" while he helps me to lie back and relax, letting him take control.

> When I do it myself, I vary pressure, speed, etc., according to what I want. It varies from one time to another, even from moment to moment. There is no way my partner can know what EXACTLY I need or want and I find it impossible to explain to him, especially as it is happening. To speak breaks concentration.

Performing Oral Sex on a Woman

For many women—at least those who have overcome their initial awkwardness about this intimate act—oral sex is more important than penetration. "Intercourse is for the man's pleasure in my mind, while cunnilingus is for my pleasure" is a common belief. One of the main reasons for this is that while it is being done *women are not expected to attend to their partner at the same time*. It is extremely important to appreciate the significance of this, especially if your partner finds it difficult to climax with intercourse. During oral sex a woman can simply lie back and enjoy it:

This is the best!!!! If I could redesign sex I'd make intercourse part of foreplay and oral sex the climax. Does that sound weird?

There's something very flattering about a man wanting to put his tongue inside you. I really enjoy my lover giving me oral sex: it can be gentle, warm and tender, but I also find it more arousing than manual sex. I also love the look of concentration on his face. However, after a while I feel almost lonely, with him down there, and have to pull him up and hold him tight.

When orally climaxing I often grab his head and push tightly towards me, it's a wonder that I don't suffocate the poor guy! Ha ha!

Oh yeah!!!! This is the absolute ultimate for me.

Despite the fact that oral sex is so immensely popular, *most* women have reservations about how they smell and what they look like "down there."

What is it about my pussy? My guy likes it. He's always going down on me. It gives me a lot of pleasure, performs a number of useful functions, and is easy to clean. It doesn't cause embarrassing protrusions when I'm feeling horny, and can be satisfied without mess in the most public places. But I'm always degrading it. I'm always thinking how lucky men are to have such a simple piece of equipment, whereas mine is this warm hole which might be fostering all manner of evils. James keeps telling me what a load of nonsense, but I keep thinking he's lying. He doesn't really like it and he's only doing it because he knows I love it—though, God knows, if that's the case, he's putting himself out much more than he really needs to.

Physically I enjoy oral sex. Psychologically no. Women have had it shoved down our throats for sooo long that we are smelly and unsightly "down there." If I had ten dollars for every deodorizing douche ad I've seen I could pay off my mortgage. Every commercial and advertisement involving your cycle is so prudish and demeaning. When someone gets you off, it's like they're really worshipping the stinkiest part of your body—or so we've been made to believe. Oral sex is therefore very difficult for me to get comfortable with, because of all those old hygiene tapes playing back in my mind.

All this is hardly surprising. Even the medical word for the vulva, "pudendum," means that "of which one ought to be ashamed." The early Christian writer Tertullian described woman as "a temple built on a sewer," although the Bible praises the region lavishly (see the Song of Solomon 4:6). Kept clean and well looked after, the vagina is a marvelous feature. Contrary to many women's fear, most men find it extremely attractive. If you've oral sex in mind, entice her into a bath or shower first. That way *she'll* know she's clean.

But how do you perform oral sex? There isn't any one way. Gentleness is the key. The lips and tongue are much softer than fingers, but still you need to make an effort not to get too carried away:

To me, my husband lacks finesse when he is giving me oral sex. I've complained often that he is hurting me with his teeth—it's too rough. I LONG just to feel hot breath on my vagina, to feel gentle caresses, to have angel kisses on my vagina's lips.

I don't always enjoy oral sex with my lover; for example, if he applies pressure with a hard rather than soft tongue, it's not comfortable at all. I have to remind him now and then about that, but he seems to forget. I think he gets too enthusiastic, but it makes me feel hostile.

Be sensitive to the woman's concerns and experiment. See how she responds. And keep it varied. Licking steadily in the same place in the same way is almost as dull for the woman as it is for you.

> Just recently I have learned a way to orgasm more quickly and intensely. While my boyfriend eats my pussy, he slowly massages my anus with a wet finger and even just barely slips the top of his finger inside my anus. It makes for an incredible orgasm!

In 1923–27 the obsessive philanderer Frank Harris published his explicit memoirs, from which the following is taken.

> "Tell me please how to give you most pleasure," I said and gently, I opened the lips of her sex and put my lips on it and my tongue against her clitoris . . . Now I varied the movement by tonguing the rest of her sex and thrusting my tongue into her as far as possible; her movements quickened and her breathing grew more and more spasmodic and when I went back to the clitoris again and took it in my lips and sucked it while pushing my forefinger back and forth into her sex, her movements became wilder and she began suddenly to cry in French, "oh, c'est fou! oh! oh!" and suddenly she lifted me up, took my head in both her hands and crushed my mouth with hers as if she wanted to hurt me.

G. Legman, in one of the most extraordinarily obsessive sex books ever written, *Oragenitalism,* quotes the following set of ways to perform oral sex on a woman, from an anonymous French book entitled *Les 32 Positions:*

> ***Clitoral Fellation.*** This is done with the tip of the tongue, in a "titillating" way. The tongue should move rapidly from right to left, or up and down, with the agility and rapidity of the finger. Women are very sensitive to this type of caress. It is to the man's interest to engage in this practice, as certain women are quite long in coming to orgasm. As soon as the woman has come, it is wise to stop this manoeuvre, for—except in rare cases—the clitoris then becomes as irritable as the man's penis does after his testicles have been emptied.
>
> ***Tonguing.*** The woman should be lying on her back, with her thighs spread. The man places his mouth on the genitals of his partner and licks her clitoris, while increasing his rhythm. The movements of his tongue finally assume the speed of the tick-tock of a clock.
>
> ***The Ice-cream Cone.*** With the thumbs and forefingers spread, place both hands at the side of the vulva, and pinch the flesh together vertically. Then press the hands together sidewise, so that the vulva becomes a sort of mound in which the clitoris is almost buried. Pass the tongue over the vulvar groove. The sensation that the clitoris feels is diminished by its wrapping of flesh, and the woman's orgasm will arrive almost imperceptibly at first but irresistibly.
>
> ***The Lollipop.*** The mouth is placed at the vaginal opening, and rubs hard against it with the flat of the tongue.
>
> ***Bird Pecking.*** The mouth is at the vulva, and the tongue travels over the inner and outer lips, which are wet with the woman's vaginal moisture. The teeth nibble at her vulva very lightly, and the tongue enters into the vagina, but the man does not attempt to suck out the moisture.

The Glutton. The man's mouth is pressed avidly to the woman's vulva, glistening with her vaginal moisture. He laps up and then swallows with relish this delicately bitter liquor, which represents her ultimate femininity and the sum of all pleasures. His tongue penetrates into the vagina, his lips kissing the woman's inner lips. (Also called *The Suction-Pump* or *Vacuum-Cleaner.*)

With a bit of imagination, there need be no end to this list, and all the various postures in which such tricks can be performed.

Important Tips for Oral and Manual Sex

1. If you're both going to do it to orgasm, let the woman climax first. Most men, despite their best intentions, lose interest once they've ejaculated, and women are acutely aware of the fact.

2. Make it absolutely clear that you enjoy what you are doing. This is especially important with oral sex.

> I needed much reassurance by my current partner that it is not an unpleasant act for him and that he is not doing it just to please me. Even still a thought at the back of my mind wonders how he could possibly love it as much as he says—yet I really enjoy him doing it to me.

> Never had an orgasm during oral sex. I don't feel comfortable—I feel as though I should come quickly so my partner doesn't have to do it for too long.

3. Remember that however much a woman is enjoying what you're doing, in order to reach orgasm she may need to stop fondling you and concentrate entirely on her own pleasure. Don't resist it. Expect it. Encourage it.

> I love manual sex physically and psychologically and feel satisfied. However, I feel selfish also as I get so wrapped up in what's being done to me. I feel I ought to be giving pleasure at the same time but I can't concentrate on both of us.

4.   Simultaneous oral stimulation for both of you—or 69—is usually most unsatisfactory for a woman. It should, to begin with, always be done with the woman lying on top, since lying underneath, upside down, with your head in a man's crotch while he goes at you at the same time is terribly uncomfortable. More than one woman has felt that her life is nearing its close when she ends up underneath the man and he pushes his penis in too far and threatens to choke her. But even when the woman is on top, 69 is rarely all it's cracked up to be. A penis is an exhausting instrument to suck, and if she's also got to think about timing her own orgasm to precede or occur simultaneously with your own—well, believe me, there are more relaxed ways of getting genital pleasure. Try it, by all means, but don't be disappointed if it doesn't have an explosive effect.

Fiddling does not have to lead to stronger things. All women enjoy occasions when it is done for its own sake, without demanding orgasm or penetration, because it is a pleasant and intimate way to pass the time. The contact is what is important, not the race for satisfaction. On such occasions, there is no reason for fiddling ever to stop, except when sleep sets in.

> Doing, a filthy pleasure is, and short;
> And done, we straight repent us of the sport
> Let us not then rush blindly on unto it,
> Like lustful beasts, that only know to do it:

For lust will languish, and that heat decay.
But thus, thus, keeping endless holiday,
Let us together, closely lie and kiss,
There is no labour, nor no shame in this;
This hath pleased, doth please, and long will please; never
Can this decay, but is beginning ever.

        —PETRONIUS ARBITER, TRANSLATED BY
        BEN JONSON

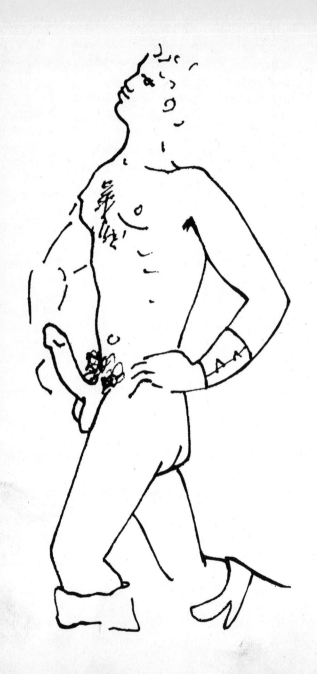

The Penis

I am a penis,
the masculine totem.
My base is a bag
that is known as the scrotum.
I'm no muscle or bone
and don't call me vein—
though I can in most men
take the place of a brain—
and I can't say my character's
lacking a stain.

—CHARLES THOMPSON,
FROM "THE PENIS POEM"

*E*arly in the morning of May 6, 1821, Professor Francesco Antommarchi entered a cottage on the northeast of the island of St. Helena brandishing a scalpel. A dozen men were standing around talking in low voices. Lying on the kitchen table between them was the freshly dead body of Napoleon Bonaparte. The professor pulled back the sheet that covered his ex-emperor's chest, took a deep breath, and sliced him open from sternum to pubis. Three hours later, the professor picked up the scalpel when nobody was watching and chopped off Mr. Bonaparte's penis as well.

The body of the greatest soldier since Hannibal lies buried in an unnamed grave; but his penis lives on. Barely an inch long, black as an ancient banana, it now rests in state on blue morocco and velvet, and belongs to the Professor and Chairman Emeritus of the Columbia University College of Physicians and Surgeons.

The monk Rasputin's appendage was also lopped off. After cuckolding half the Russian imperial court, the smelly owner was poisoned with an enormous dose of cyanide, shot, raped, castrated, and finally, proving too durable for such moderate measures, drowned under ice. Rasputin's withered penis is thirteen inches long, and was last seen in 1968 in a polished wooden box in a Parisian lady's bedroom.

Somewhere between these two mummified extremes lies the typical prick, a flaccid bit of sponge between three and four and a half inches long, although, as any bathing belle can testify, swimming in a cold sea will shrink it to nothing. Physical strain can have the same effect and old age diminishes the poor thing still further, both in dimension and vitality—"the useless rag of manhood flopping against the thigh," as one novelist has it. (But take heart, many male members are vigorous at seventy and I have just met someone who was conceived when his father was seventy-nine.)

However, the big question in every man's mind is not how

l

  o

    n

    g

                    G

                   N

                  O

is it dangling, but how **L** will it become when erect?

Limp size is misleading, so ignore the critical ogling from the man in the next urinal. Small ones expand more than large ones. Most erect penises are between four and eight inches in length, with six and a bit inches the average. Watching *King Kong and the Six Panting Virgins* would make anyone feel that six inches scarcely qualified as a protrusion at all, but saw your old school ruler in two and you'll see that half a foot is nothing to be ashamed of. Remember, the resting vagina is only three to four inches deep. For those keen to be precise, here's a table.

small:	Less than five inches
average:	Six inches
large:	Over seven inches
enormous:	Nine inches plus

Other classifications are quite possible, however. The *Kama Sutra* (Indian, first century A.D.) divides the penis into three types: hare, bull, and horse. The hare is less than five inches with sweet semen; the bull is up to seven inches; the horse, up to ten inches with semen that is copious and salty. *Amanga Ranga,* another Indian work, from the sixteenth century, adopts a prophetic approach to the problem: a thin penis means the owner will be lucky; a long one, that he will be poor; a thick one, distressed; and any man with a very small passion probe will be a ruler of the land. No prizes for guessing which type the author had.

One must also keep in mind the number of penises a man has. The Egyptian god Osiris is often depicted as a fiery bull with three copulatory instruments, but such penile oddities are not confined to fiction. Mortal men with *two* functioning penises and *two sets* of testicles are well documented. Another curiosity is the autosexual, typified by an inmate of a Soviet labor camp in the 1960s. He could bend his penis between his legs, penetrate his own anus, and by contracting his rectal muscles satisfy himself, which he regularly did. This extraordinary fellow was intensely narcissistic and withdrawn, and refused to have any contact with other prisoners. Photographs of him in his bizarre act of masturbation—which many men fantasize about, if only for the convenience of it—were circulated throughout the camp as pornography.

I don't suppose anybody has stepped forward to claim the *Guinness Book of World Records* prize for the smallest prick in existence; the largest that I have come across (not personally, you understand) was the unofficial world record, circa 1970, of fourteen inches long and three in diameter. The biggest (real) limp one is even larger, and belongs to Whistling Charlie of Hollywood, who displays it on a silver platter at parties. Alas, this organ is so large that it has never managed an erection. Johnny Wadd, hero of such educational classics as *Deep Throat,* had a twelve-incher (and insisted he had a perfectly ordinary sex life), but no man on earth can compete with a walrus . . . his organ is two feet long, contains a bone, and is so sturdy that Eskimos sometimes use it as a war club.

What Do Women Think about Penises?

"Many females," wrote Professor Kinsey after interviewing several thousand of us, "consider [the male organ] ugly and repulsive in appearance . . . and the sight of it may actually inhibit their erotic responses."

Oh dear.

Not what you want to hear.

But it's no good hoping that women have changed their opinions since that time. We haven't.

The male member is not a thing of beauty. It serves a delightful purpose, but on the purely aesthetic plane a penis is not a prizewinner. A cynical female friend of mine describes it as "a crinkly, hairy bag with a scrunched-up tube on the end, which occasionally becomes engorged with blood, and has a tendency to smell unless the floppy bit of skin at the end is cut off." Certainly Freud must have been suffering one of his cocaine dreams when he said women envy the male organ (what they more likely envy is its ability to climax easily). It comes as no surprise to us that eight times as many transsexuals are men wanting to become female than vice versa. Whenever I see a set of male organs I am irrepressibly reminded of the school pottery class, where we were told always to mold from the original lump of clay, and never never to stick bits on a piece of sculpture. I just *know* that if you put a man into a pottery oven his sexual organs will drop off.

In the words of the ever-trenchant British columnist Julie Burchill, "I have never met a woman who contemplated the extension without a degree of horror."

> The whole thing's a bit ridiculous. There you are. In front of you stands the nude man, your one-night stand, your passing fancy, your lover, your husband . . . and he's got this funny thing with droopy bits sticking out in front of him about halfway up, where his legs meet.

> When I meet a new man at a party, after I've drunk a little and we start making out, I always put my hand down his pants in the dark. I like to know what's coming.

> It absolutely beats me why men are obsessed with the things—so proud of them. Always strutting about the bedroom with a hard-on. They look so ridiculous!

> When a man undresses for a woman for the first time, it's an anxious moment for both of you. I'm terrified it's going to be really ugly, or a funny shape, that I'll be embarrassed for him and repelled myself.

> I remember the very first time I saw a penis, I couldn't believe it, it was so big and red and peculiar. I was

about seven and I watched my father going to the bathroom. I was fascinated and horrified at this huge thing
being sort of unwrapped. Mom was so clean and
smooth.

The angle kills me. Exactly like a flagpole . . . I hung a
flag on my boyfriend's dick once.

Sniffy, mocking, incredulous, or contorted with hysterical
laughter women may be, yet when we're all alone and need to
find a penis substitute we soon realize just how well designed
the real thing is. Hairbrush handles and candles are too hard,
pencils too thin; a cucumber isn't bad providing it's been
warmed up in the microwave. Cynthia has experimented and
discovered that a "banana isn't really straight enough" but a car-
rot with a condom on is "beautiful." If it's simply the feel of it
and not the *use,* there's only one thing that really approximates
an erect penis, i.e., firm yet not unyielding, and warm withal—
and that's a ten-foot python (a shorter serpent hasn't got the
requisite girth).

Aside from lack of beauty, a key complaint women have
about the penis is the number of men who use it as a power
symbol. It's hard for us to see an unfamiliar lover's erection
without feeling a touch wary. Is he going to get carried away
with the grandeur of his instrument and give us a difficult,
painful, or tedious time? What rights does he imagine it gives
him over us? Will this be erotic intercourse, or just an uncomfortable, soulless form of masturbation for the man? The Asmat
and Auyu tribes of southern New Guinea put on a display that
is a woman's idea of a nightmare. When visitors arrive they run
about with erect penises, grasping and rubbing them, spreading
their thighs, and thrusting out their pelvises. They also do it in
a thunderstorm or if a house catches fire.

The sight of an erect penis does not send women into immediate rapturous arousal. If it did, flashers, who like to shock

and outrage, would be permanently out of business. (Female readers: next time you are flashed at, lean forward, peer closely, and say in a loud voice, "Hhhmmmm, looks like a penis only smaller.") Women don't find the thing sexy per se, nor men's hairy tops of thighs and dangly parts. We want them covered up until the right moment. Only in a sexy situation with a gorgeous fellow can a penis transform itself into something attractive.

Men concentrate on size, but for women shape, color, texture, circumference, whether it's circumcised or not, the way it hangs, how it stands, the shape of the head, the straightness of the shaft, are just as important penile considerations.

I like a pale penis, straight and clean-looking.

A mottled, drunken penis has a jolly, well-used look. Pale pricks are priggish. Give me a drunken philanderer.

I love the shaft. Straight and almost smooth. If you run your hand down a prick there are these tiny little bumps.

There are nice pricks in the world and there are ugly ones. More ugly than beautiful, that's for sure. You don't have to be promiscuous to know that, just buy *Playgirl*!

Not particular, just so it works.

I'm fussy about balls. The best? Rounded, high-up, tight—very sexy. Nice to touch too. Mmmmmmm.

I like hanging testicles. I can get my mouth round them.

You know what I like [in the way of male organs]? Stud farm bulls. Brawn and muscle, and great pendulous balls and prick. And the ring through their nose gives them such a cute-looking face. And shoulders—God, I can hardly pass a farmyard without fainting. I used to visit the local cattle market every week when I was a teenager. How can I take a man seriously after that?

Practical features are more important than mere looks: "I'll tell you a secret," writes Zara. "Long hanging testicles are no beauties. But they feel great. Get the guy to fuck you slowly and feel them bumping against you." Of the two basic shapes, the Straight and the Banana, some women are strongly partisan and contend that you get a better class of satisfaction with one or the other. "I have this theory," writes Geraldine, "that a Banana gives better friction on the clitoris because of the slight curve."

Another very important quality of a penis is how long it stays erect after ejaculation. Those that detumesce quickly need fast work if you're using a condom, to prevent the semen spilling out. Greatly prized is the penis that remains hard for five or more minutes after ejaculation, thus allowing tardy females to catch up on their satisfaction.

Women divide on the subject of circumcision. I'm fervently in favor, and was most annoyed to learn that, although the future British king has been done, the Princess of Wales refused to let the future future king be seen to. Circumcision confers several advantages. The penis looks smooth and aesthetic, it will be cleaner, and some women insist it lasts longer. A man who's been circumcised is used to things rubbing against his penis head and is, as a consequence, less sensitive during intercourse. Uncircumcised men need to make a great effort to wash thoroughly: there's a subtle difference between being clean enough for a nose that's two feet distant (your own) and one at point-blank range. I was told by a medical man that the ultra-smooth skin cut from penis circumcision is used in facial plastic surgery. I still haven't decided if he was pulling my leg or not.

Obviously penises vary enormously from man to man; what is more remarkable is how much one penis can vary from day to day. Observant women can tell, often to within an hour or so, when lover-boy last climaxed. "If he's masturbated, I know by how it feels," remarked several women. Addie knew her husband was having an affair because, although he was scrupulously careful about hiding every detail, his own penis gave him away. "It just wasn't as big as it used to be. Whenever we made love it felt different from how it used to, as if it were working on 70 percent capacity." I got together with a group of experts and we came up with the Four Degrees (of erectness in a penis):

1.   The Ramrod Maximum length and sexually very sensitive. Almost a twitchy feel, as if the semen might shoot out any moment. The sort of penis that invites a blow job, because you have the pleasure of his pleasure but you know he won't be able to last long ("Blow jobs are *tiring*").

2.   The Good and Ready Full, taut, but not shiny-taut. This is ideal for penetration because it'll last quite a bit longer than state 1.

3.   The Heavy Flopper This is a popular penis state. You lose nothing on the size, but it's a laid-back penis. Instead of standing to arms, it's cool, reclining slightly, and unthreatening. It feels heavy in your hand because it's not self-supporting.

4.   The Only Just A suspicious state if you and he have not had sex recently: either he's very tired or someone else has made him tired. On the positive side, this state of penis often inspires a woman to begin on oral sex. It gets him going and it's easier to perform when he's small. For men with erection difficulties see chapter 7.

Some women, I regret to say, would be quite happy if they never saw another penis:

Oh, I'm no nun, I love men and I love sex. But tongues and hands can do all the work—who needs a great stiff rod poking away at you and making you sore?

There's a category of men I call Willy Wavers—the kind who in bed are always making you do something to their prick—always nudging you with it.

I can get off on being masturbated, with his hand, or the arm of my teddy bear—I'm quite happy and relaxed until I have to start thinking about *that thing*.

It's not just that it doesn't do anything for me, but I always have to attend to it, rubbing, sucking, oh God! They talk about women as sex objects. Penises turn some men into *objects*. I'd much rather have the whole of him. I love the way he talks, his eyes, his hands. Yet so often he reduces himself to that silly little thing between his legs.

Is Penis Size Important?

The real question is, important to whom?

To men, size is very, very important. Julian, an architect, thirty-two years old, six and a quarter inches, and a perfectly average, well-adjusted, unmacho specimen of manhood, revealed to me that his life had been blighted by concerns about the dimension of his organ:

Size was everything. From time immemorial the penis has been considered a symbol of fertility, and the last thing you want as the symbol of your procreative powers is a matchstick. At school you were always comparing with the other boys, and those that were worried were the last ones to dash in and out of the shower or they stood awkwardly, half-facing the wall, and using their hands to cover themselves. It wasn't even as if we even knew how to have sex. It was just part of the equipment of being a man. More than that, it was fundamental to your future dominance in the adult world. A big cock could make up for bad football skills, bad grades, recurrent acne . . .

Alan, a mechanic, twenty-eight years old, eight inches (so I'm told), and as cocksure as anybody I've met, confessed the following fraught story:

When I was a kid I worried over my little thing all the time. It wasn't hairy, then it got hairy, but it didn't seem to get any bigger, and I knew for a fact that a real man has one that hangs to his knees. There was a school physical. I knew that one of the things the doctor would be checking was that I had two testicles, and I also knew that I only had one. No amount of exploration could discover the other one. Perhaps they'd fused together because I'd been wearing tight jeans. I knew the doctor would exclaim out loud in front of the rest of the school that Alan has only got one ball. So I ran away from school and refused to go back. It was one long litany of impending disaster as far as my dick was concerned. After I'd found the other testicle, I began to worry about the shape. It looked too curvy. And about the length again—definitely undersized. Already thirteen and only three inches to show for it. And then about the erection angle. Surely nothing that went up that far would be any use to anybody. A proper penis obviously poked straight out in front, whereas mine was up like a Heil Hitler! And then about the length once more . . .

Andy, a scientific photographer, twenty-five years old, five and three-fifths inches, pursued Sally patiently for months and at long last captured her interest. She lured him back to the bedroom where the long-awaited consummation was obviously to happen. "This was going to be sheer bliss," he thought.

After a delicious meal and lots of wine it was lights down low time. I went to the bathroom and started getting ready, when suddenly . . . panic! I can't explain it. I thought "She's not going to like my prick. It's too small." It looked smaller than ever, like a dot at the top of my legs. I tried kneading it. I tried running it under hot water. I laid it on the heater. I found something that promised to enlarge my breasts in Sally's medicine cabinet, so I squeezed some of that on and after five minutes it got tingly. Next it went bright red and hot and in my drunken state I thought it was a great improvement. When I came back in Sally switched on the light. My prick was puffy and purple. She took one look and shrieked blue murder so the whole apartment building came running.

Size matters. No amount of sweet-talking is going to convince men otherwise. A guy with a five-incher might come to terms with it, and be the best bed fighter in the world, but, if he ever gets jealous, you can bet your last penny that he'll be convinced his rival's main attraction is that he has a bigger, thicker, more satisfying organ. A man with a small penis cannot be anything other than constantly aware of it. So great, indeed, is the male concern about size that in Asia and Africa there have been periodic epidemics of "Koro," the groundless conviction that one's penis is shrinking and going to disappear. Whole communities wake up one morning convinced that their manhood is being gobbled up. One doctor recorded 4,500 cases of this distressing condition in his region.

Does Size Matter to Women?

> Women talk at great length about penises. Get a bunch of girls together and there's no stopping them. Out come all the penis stories they know—measurements and all the rest.
>
> —MARGARET POWELL, *THE TREASURE UPSTAIRS*

The "treasure" does not refer to a naked superstud waiting in the bedroom. Margaret Powell's book is about life as a servant in the 1920s and contains plenty of references to penises, which shows how prevalent female interest in the male member has always been. If men could listen in to all this woman talk they'd know at once that the two most popular phallic phallusies are contradictory:

Phallusy No. 1: The Larger the Prick the More Satisfied the Woman

Phallusy No. 2: Women Don't Care about Penis Size

Most men adhere to one or other of these two extreme beliefs. The sensitive sex therapist tells the world that a little ding-a-ling is to be treasured provided it's well used. Masters and Johnson concluded, after much careful work, that size makes no difference at all to female satisfaction—but since many men have difficulty satisfying a woman in the first place, this conclusion doesn't mean very much. David Reuben, another self-appointed male "authority" on women's innermost concerns, gives the following simplistic reason for why women don't care about dimension:

> Almost every aspect of orgiastic sensation in women is concentrated in the accessible genital structures, that is the clitoris, labia, and related areas. This includes the

lower one-third of the vagina, in easy reach of nearly every post-adolescent penis. In sexual intercourse, as in every artistic endeavour, it is quality not quantity that counts.

Julie Burchill, on the other hand, announces gleefully: "98 percent of women interviewed by Shere Hite declared themselves 'disappointed' with heterosex. If men are equal, and technique can be learned, why should this be so? The answer is probably that 98 percent of American men have a small penis."

Don't trust any of them. The therapists are scared they'll mess up the male ego and lose clients. Burchill's after notoriety and the pleasure of giving nasty, small-penised misogynists a good rattling down. I understand her temptation, but she'll only make them even nastier.

Now you're going to get the truth:

SIZE DOES *MATTER*.

Let's actually ask some ordinary women. We'll begin with me. Rachel, what's your opinion of small penises?

"Hmmmm, I must admit I've seen one or two itty-bitty ones in my time and I wasn't thrilled. That hogwash of David Reuben's doesn't take account of the all-important *psychology* of sexual excitement. The *idea* of what's happening to you in sex is one of the best parts—for women especially. It explains why few of us are likely to get an orgasm from a brilliantly techniqued fellow we don't like. And though the upper part of the vagina may not have as many nerves, you can damn well feel a penis up there, and I like the feeling. No, small ones are not for me. My preference is for a pale, smooth, circumcised seven-incher, I'm quite specific about that." Thank you, Rachel. Very nicely put.

Liz Barnes and her boyfriend James were recently featured in *Woman's Own*. Liz was unequivocal about his four-inch penis: "The first time I saw James naked I cringed—his penis was so thin and puny that it made me feel sick." So one day she stomped out of the house and refused to come back unless he made it bigger. Six weeks and $5,000 of plastic surgery later, James was two inches longer and two and a half inches bigger in circumference. Liz is now happy: "The difference it's made to our love life is incredible," she exclaims. "Many women have breast implants to please their partners, so why shouldn't I ask James to have his willy enlarged?"

The Hung Jury Club in America was founded for women who prefer penises eight inches or longer, and they get some absolute whoppers. There is no sweet-talking around the fact that just as men have breast size preferences, a lot of women prefer a certain length of penis (though it doesn't necessarily mean we won't tolerate any other).

> Does size matter? Course it does! Don't you believe any of those ridiculous myths that state that women don't mind what size your equipment is. I sometimes think that all that virginity nonsense was maintained simply so that it saved men the indignity of having their willies compared.

> You can feel it, of course you can. They say a woman is elastic, but she's elastic the other way: she can take something huge, but that doesn't mean she likes something small.

> You know what kind of man's really worth holding on to? A man with a good average-sized prick, somewhere between six and seven inches. Why? For peace, that's why. 'Cause a little prick and he's always grizzling about it and

wanting reassurance. With a whopper, he's forever boasting and not bothering with other techniques. Christ!

Size is unimportant in terms of performance, but it matters aesthetically. If the man's penis is proportionate to his body, that's okay—smaller penis on a smaller guy and vice versa.

Show me a frigid woman and, nine times out of ten, I'll show you a little man. Face it: every girl wants one, and every man does too; no one, given the chance, would *choose* the small model. If it's so good, why is the dildo industry built on twelve-inchers? Why do rock stars stuff handkerchiefs down their pants rather than bind down the offending object? And why are condoms never marked Small, Medium and Large but Large, Jumbo and Super Jumbo? Because instinct admits to what indoctrination cannot swallow.

How big is big? More than eight inches. More than eleven can be problematic. But not half as problematic as less than seven!

—JULIE BURCHILL, GETTING EVER MORE
CARRIED AWAY

For a second type of woman size really is irrelevant. Mr. Thomas is a glassblower: very large in the chest, with a voice that could rattle the rafters of St. Paul's, but rather less than monumental down below. His wife, fifty-three, doesn't mind a bit. "He's a lusty man and he throws me around, which I enjoy. As long as he goes at me with energy I'm happy. I love to rest on his big chest and feel his hips at me. Completely satisfied." Writes Paula, "I'd never want a man to worry about his size or even think about it, if possible."

[Ian] always thinks he's not big enough to satisfy me. I wouldn't care if "my friend" was the size of a pencil, I only want him, he only has to touch me and he can drive me mad with desire . . .

If it's attached to a nice head and torso I'll forget the weeniness. I'm generous.

I don't mind that Yosuah has a very small one because it's very thick. I call it his Cumberland sausage. It stretches me.

Size is unimportant. I can take all sizes as long as he uses it well. All women are like that. They think they couldn't have this or that but they could and would be happy with it if they were happy with the man.

And then there are those who are positively *anti* big ones. "You know, the young men seem to be getting bigger and bigger," remarked a prostitute in 1959. "It must be the Welfare State. I hate it though; it splits me." Moral: listen to the professionals. Harold Robbins didn't when he wrote *The Betsy,* a favorite piece with writers of sex textbooks, used to illustrate what nonsensical ideas some authors have about women's lust for size:

Gently her fingers opened his union suit and he sprang out at her like an angry lion from its cage. Carefully she peeled back his foreskin, exposing his red and angry glans, and took him in both hands, one behind the other as if she were grasping a baseball bat. She stared at it in wonder. *"C'est formidable. Un vrai canon . . ."*

She moaned in pain and writhed, her pelvis suddenly arching and thrusting toward him. Then he entered her again.

"Mon Dieu!" she cried, the tears springing into her eyes. *"Mon Dieu!"* She began to climax almost before he was fully inside her. Then she couldn't stop them,

one coming rapidly after the other as he slammed into her with the force of the giant body press she had seen working in his factory . . .

One wonders if Mr. Robbins has ever been with a woman at all, that he could dream up such nonsense. A punch against the ovaries with a baseball bat–size truncheon of hard flesh is extremely nasty. And women have never climaxed like this in the history of humankind, provoked by the sight of size alone, in the midst of agony. Pain is pain is pain.

In conclusion, I'll quote from a letter I got from a woman in Glasgow, Scotland.

I seem to get the freaks. One will be an incher and the next a foot. Of the two, I prefer the foot to look at and the incher to use. But over the years I've got pretty adept at exploiting both. Taking the foot first. I can't accommodate it. I like to feel it inside me, but only part of the way, and then I have to be on top where I can control how much penetration there is. If I'm underneath I feel nervous. There's always a chance he might forget his promise not to keep forcing, although you can prevent this by keeping your hand round the base or making him put on one of those things sex shops sell. But the main trouble is that whichever way you choose, there isn't much pressure on your clitoris. The small penis however doesn't give you so much to squeeze on, but it does mean that he's right there on top of you and not pushed down a few inches. His pubic bone is in the right place to give the right pressure. Also I've noticed that small men tend to fall into two types—the really bad and the very good lovers. In my experience, small penised men tend to be better lovers than normal sized ones.

What Can I Do with a Penis That Is Too Small?

You have three options: (a) concentrate on other attractions, (b) exercise, and (c) enlarge. Taking them in order:

(a) Other Attractions: Most women are prepared to accept and love a small penis, provided the owner makes up the difference by top-notch lovemaking, e.g.:

> **She:** Ha! ha! ha! What's that?!
>
> **He:** My dart of happiness. My drumstick of passion. It beats for three hours, to a perfect rhythm.
>
> **She:** Right! Get it over here on the double!

His nice straightforward approach is good too: neither bumptious nor apologetic. In fact, it's often the attitude that goes with a small one, rather than the thing itself that puts a woman off. Relax, forget the blessed item, and recollect that she is certainly self-conscious about her bottom.

Bad lovers are a thousand times more common than undersized organs, and a small penis has plenty of potential. "It's four inches, although it's quite thick for the size," writes the astonishingly frank Mr. Dover. "It makes you hate at times. You can go down two roads. Either you indulge the hate, and decide all women are whores. Or you can fight it. A small organ does not mean women don't want you . . . It definitely does not mean you can't satisfy your partner. You've got to learn skills. To my enormous surprise, I've now developed a reputation as a good lover. Small dick, but a good lay. Women hate a big penis if it's got a goat for a man on the other end." Hear, hear.

(b) Exercise: Not you, her. There aren't any penis building-up exercises for men because *the penis isn't a muscle*. But women can do Kegel exercises to strengthen their pubococcygeal (PC) muscles and thus improve their grip on and pleasure from your little prize. These exercises really work. See chapter 7 for a full description of the Kegels.

(c) Enlarge: "Penis enhancement" surgery is a growing business in America. One surgeon claims to have performed 70 percent of all such operations—fourteen a day on males aged from sixteen to seventy-eight. For around $6,000 he offers extra length or extra girth. Both are very delicate operations, and, as with breast augmentation, it should always be the owner's decision, not the partner's. Six of this surgeon's customers are currently claiming medical malpractice: one became impotent, another disfigured, a third suffered gangrene of the penis and scrotum, and a number of patients' organs got shorter. If you value your manhood, don't believe extravagant claims and check up very carefully about what's involved.

Apart from surgery, nothing makes a penis larger: pills, potions, or any other gizmo. But what about the penis enlarger machines advertised in men's magazines? After reading a manufacturer's warning that purple spots were likely to appear upon the penis, I certainly wasn't going to risk my boyfriend's precious parts on one of those. Michael Castleman, an American expert on men's sexual difficulties, writes that the gadget is "as simple as it is useless . . . The bottom line is that penis enlargers are a fraud." The purple spots are due to hemorrhaging: the vacuum forces so much blood into the penis that some of the capillaries burst. The whole idea is most distasteful!

What Can I Do with a Penis That Is Too Large?

How you deal with a too-large organ is vitally important from the point of view of a woman's comfort. The French have a useful device called a bourrelet, a small silk pad with a hole in the middle that is attached by two ribands to the woman's thighs: the penis enters her through the hole, and thus only the desired amount of penetration is allowed. It would be far easier to put a doughnut-shaped pad around the base of your penis. No doubt such devices are advertised in sex aids catalogs, but you could make one easily. Cut two ring doughnut shapes out of a piece of old sheet, the inner circle being of the same diameter as your erect member. Sew together, and stuff with suitable fluff.

Always make absolutely certain that your lover is fully aroused before penetration, because only then will her vaginal canal be ready for you. Even then you must inch in with caution, letting her control the rate. Pillows placed under her back will allow her to raise her hips into the most comfortable position.

Can a Woman Tell Your Size without Undressing You?

Naturally. A man with more than one rottweiler has less than five inches. Add tinted glasses and a low-slung car from Italy, 0 to 95 in four seconds, and he loses another inch. The gray matter of this sort of man is also smaller. How else could he have reached manhood without noticing that the speed limit is 65 mph?

Physically, there is no correlation between overall body size and penis dimension. Gorillas have tiny pricks. The friendly seaside barnacle, on the other hand, has a penis thirty times the length of its body. Among humans, some people doggedly adhere to the importance of fingers and noses as size indicators.

A maiden's mouth shows what's the make of her chose;
And man's mentula one knows by the length of his nose;
And the eyebrows disclose how the lower wig grows.
—SIR RICHARD BURTON

Despite the numerous studies disproving any connection between general body build and penile endowment (the largest penis in one study belonged to a man of five foot seven), I have found nothing on the penis/nose or penis/hands and feet correlation. If anybody has any evidence either way (not physical, if you please!), I'd be interested to hear it.

Are there racial variations? Political correctness makes researchers nowadays insist that all differences are fictional. Women gossiping together tend to disagree, though their findings must remain a secret. And geographical differences? The following, using a botanical metaphor, is from a book published in 1793 (*The School of Venus*):

> [The penis] is produced in most countries, tho' it thrives more in some than in others, where it also increases to a larger Size. The Height here in England rarely passes nine or eleven inches, and that chiefly in Kent; whereas in Ireland it comes to far greater dimensions; is so good, that many of the Nations entirely subsist upon it and, when transplanted, have been sometimes known to raise good Houses with single plants of the sort.

Kit Schwartz, in his book *The Male Member*, remarks that "many nations require condoms to measure up to . . . specifications before allowing entry. This is especially true when it comes to length. For instance, the condom in Britain is taller than those used by Yanks, and the Yanks' is taller than the Japanese. Surprisingly, the Yank is too tall for entry into Hungary and, staggeringly, the Hungarians are so shortsighted as to admit it."

The Penis Rubbed

Performing manual sex on men is not popular with women. It's hard work, and because we're built so differently we worry that we're doing it wrong. How hard should we press? Which rhythm? How much lubrication is comfortable? Where to get all that lubrication from? Men who like having it performed should give plenty of encouragement when the partner does it right. If she does it wrong, instead of the crushing comment, "Not like that!" be tactful. For example: "Mmmm, I like that [a slight untruth] but up a bit more." Gently guiding her hands to the right place is best of all.

> I tend to get aroused by a very gentle touch and find it hard to believe when my boyfriend wants a hard grip. I keep stopping and asking him, "Are you sure this is right?"

> I find it difficult to keep going. It often takes a long time for a man to come this way, and it can be very exhausting on the arm. And, to add fuel to the flames, men having this done to them tend to forget about the woman. So there you are getting more and more achy while he is smiling idiotically. Then I get really angry and resentful.

> Two or three minutes is a long time to the penis rubber. Your arm aches like hell. It's so exhausting. Men don't realize because when they do it to themselves they're naturally at the right angle. And where's your reward?

> I only ever give a hand job if it's an easy way to get out of an awkward situation.

> I remember with acute embarrassment the day I first held a penis. I was sixteen years old, at a party, and while kissing with a man I put my hand down his pants. My rings caught in his pubic hair.

If your partner is absolutely hopeless, suggest you masturbate in front of her. Some women find it very sexy. Other women feel that manual sex is rather squalid. It suggests dingy corners in Times Square, and quickies in the car with a streetwalker. For Francie, a thirty-eight-year-old photographer, it is unpleasantly reminiscent of early sexual encounters:

> God, I remember my first encounter with a real live penis. I was working in a disco, seventeen years old and pretty naïve. This guy took me home. I really liked him but he was about thirty-five. We lay on the bed, caressing and such. Now I guess as I was so young and virginal he didn't dare have the responsibility of fucking me, but he wanted something. So he took out his prick and put it in my hand. I was shocked: it looked so big and red. I just sort of vaguely fiddled with it, not having a clue really. And he says: "Let me give you a tip. You should rub this." But he obviously realized I was hopeless so he just kept rubbing it himself until he ejaculated—all over my new jacket. It wasn't pretty.

What women do enjoy is gently fondling their partner's penis; the pleasurable sensation of fingers sliding around it, or softly up and down. It is when there is intense pressure to bring the man to orgasm that manual sex can become a burden.

The Penis Sucked

With many women, performing oral sex is much more popular than manual sex, *provided the circumstances are right.* Just as well, since it seems that every other man's fantasy is a woman who'll give him a blow job three times a day and never complain. The "right circumstances" are when the service is offered, not demanded. And when there is mutual respect and affection.

> My favorite part of lovemaking is when I take the penis in my right hand and lower my mouth towards it. I flick my tongue across the top of it, then gently around the

ridge, wetting it all over. Now I use it like a lipstick, as if I'm making up my lips, smoothing it from side to side, up into the cupid's bow and gliding on along. And now the bottom lip . . . mmmm. I love that feeling. It's what pricks were invented for. But they must must must be circumcised.

I like it extremely [actually spelled, in her enthusiasm, esteemly], I can't have sex without oral sex. That's part of foreplay. I love the taste, feel and smell of the flesh while doing oral sex. The taste is hot and salty from the sweat and juices from the penis. I love the feel of two bodies intertwining, hands and tongue exploring every inch of each other's bodies. The smell of hot flesh, clean but sweaty bodies, the smell of each other's juices. I'm a walking G-zone and ABSOLUTELY love sex.

Women particularly enjoy the emotional intimacy of it:

When I have a love affair I always consider carefully— and remember afterwards—the moment I first take his penis in my mouth. And, more importantly, the first time he ejaculates in my mouth.

I think I enjoy giving him oral sex more than I like receiving it. I like the feeling of control and the noises he makes.

In a way the act has taken the place of ordinary penetration as symbolic of love and intimacy.

But it's not all roses. Nutty book though it is, *The Dieter's Guide to Weight Loss during Sex* remarks acutely that, whereas cunnilingus burns up fifteen calories, fellatio uses up thirty: "It uses more muscles, especially those of the neck, hands, and eyes." I recommend that a man perform oral sex for five minutes without stopping on an unpeeled banana without marking the skin. It'll make you a more tolerant specimen in the future! Penises, even the smallest ones, can never be small enough when it comes to sucking a man. It is very tiring on the old jaws to have a five-inch-circumference pink piston in your mouth. You are more likely to get oral sex for longer if you encourage your partner not just to suck but also to lick the object and use her hands at the same time. That way the process is much less tiring.

I will only do it when I want to and I have to be relaxed and feel in control and that I won't get gagged to death. I can't handle his penis deep in my throat.

Oral sex is a double bind. The longer you go on with a blow job, the more painful it gets and the harder to keep going. But the closer he gets to ejaculation, the meaner it seems to stop.

I enjoy sucking my husband only in a playful way, not letting the penis far into my mouth, because I find it very uncomfortable and it makes me retch at times. Sometimes if very roused I can enjoy taking it in further but I am then afraid I will bite by accident. I just don't feel skilled in this activity.

First and foremost sucking him off is damned uncomfortable to do. I wonder if heterosexual men have any idea of just what hard work it is, keeping your mouth open over six inches, wide enough not to let your teeth scrape and long enough for him to come? It's agony. Your jaw aches.

And the mouthful of semen? I don't know many women who actually enjoy swallowing it, though they like to do it for the sake of closeness.

I just shut my eyes and swallow without tasting. Then I go straight to clean my teeth. That way if you're slick and skillful you can get away with barely tasting it.

I dislike the taste but love the smell of it, that sweet bedroom smell. Semen is like cigarette smoke: sweet and heady on the first puff, disgusting when it's stale.

Semen, however, is nutritious, and nutrition is fattening. I remember my first year at college. My next-door neighbor in the dorm was a charming woman who was having an intense affair, and trying to lose weight. One afternoon, half an hour after I had seen her lover arrive, she burst into my room very tipsy and demanded to know how many calories semen contained. "Twenty-seven," I answered sweetly.

A number of female fantasies involve Niagara-style gushes of semen:

My favorite thing? To have him fuck me, him on top, in and out. And then at the last minute he pulls out of me and squirts his stuff all over me, my cunt, my clitoris, my spread legs.

In my fantasy, I'm asleep in bed, very demure in a brushed nylon nightie. You know, a homely type, a little plump. I hear a noise. A burglar is in the other room. He comes into my room and I wake up. He's very polite: absolutely no physical threat at all, no violence, nothing like that. Only polite humiliation.

He pulls back the bedclothes, looks me all over and tells me, "Excuse me, I have to do this." He now unzips his pants, takes out his prick and begins to masturbate. I'm sitting up in bed meanwhile, can't help watching him. He's polite and nice, but doing what he wants. He can't control himself. So I watch him stroking, up and down. Even though I'm a virgin I can tell he's getting closer. Suddenly he says to me, "I'm so sorry, but I have to do this." Very polite still. He leans over and unbuttons my nightie to the waist. My large breasts are revealed. He kneels over me on the bed and strokes and strokes—and squirts his juice all over me. A blob goes on my mouth and chin.

He apologizes politely and leaves.

That is my fantasy. And yet I am not overjoyed when my husband ejaculates all over me in bed.

If it's a new partner, be careful where you deposit your semen. Ejaculation, almost more than any other aspect of ordinary sex, occupies an uncertain territory between being utterly, wantonly sexy and downright tacky (in both senses of the word). Misplaced semen can in an instant turn a romantic passion into a sordid screw, not to mention ruining clothes and carpets.

All in all the golden rule of oral sex is: **Don't Insist.** Some women hate the very idea of it. As for the rest of us, there's a world of difference between the pleasure of offering to suck a lover's penis, and the complete and utter turn-off of feeling obliged to do it.

Finally, here is an Anglo-Saxon riddle:

Swings by his thigh a thing most magical!
Below the belt, beneath the folds
Of his clothes it hangs, a hole in its front end,
Stiff-set and stout, but swivels about.
Levelling the head of this hanging instrument,
Its wielder hoists his hem above the knee:
It is his will to fill a well-known hole
That it fits fully when at full length.
He has often filled it before. Now he fills it again.

Think you know the answer? Now check: it's the same as the sixth and seventh words of the next to last paragraph on page 108.

7

Penetration

*E*very day, around the world, there are 100 million acts of sexual intercourse. That's over 1.5 million quarts of semen resulting in 910,000 conceptions, 150,000 abortions, and 350,000 cases of sexually transmitted diseases per day.

Excuse me while I faint.

As sexual intercourse is usually taken to mean penetration, let's begin with the organ that makes it possible . . .

The Vagina

> One other thing there was, black-fringed, grasping, dainty and fresh, but the name of that I may not tell. Words fail to describe the charm of so beauteous a vision.
>
> —*THE GOLDEN LOTUS*

In these cautious days, it has become commonplace to point out that the few current euphemisms and slang terms for the vagina tend to be either abusive, passive, or unpublishable. "Cunt," for example, was banned from print from 1300 until the middle of the twentieth century, and it's still considered more foul than "fuck."

But we have not always been so linguistically impoverished. In a good dictionary of slang you'll find about twice as many terms for the vagina as you will for the penis. To name a few: claff, kitty, madge, star, oven, valve, cup, bell, chum, kaze, quem, quiff, quimmy, quin, surf, bazoo, keifer, fanny, beaver, twat, pleasure house, marble arch, leak, mate, temple of low men, temple of Venus, upright wink, forecastle, valley of decision, bearded lady, gasp and grunt, old ding, penis(!), old mossyface, intercural trench, belly-dale, gentleman's pleasure garden, hole of holes, Eve's custom house, spender, bawdy monosyllable, snatch box, fly catcher, skin the puzzle, crinkum-crankum, eye that weeps most when best pleased, shaft-companion, yeast powder biscuit, hamburger, cream jug, sugar doughnut, bit on a fork, fanny artful, tirly-whirly, box unseen, Lapland, manhole, jiggumbob, jewel, mother of all saints, mother of all souls, cockshire, rob-the-ruffian, tail, tail end, and the end.

"Vagina" comes from the Latin word for sheath, and the flexibility of it is astonishing. In the resting state it is three to four inches long and flattened, yet it can accommodate a baby's head. Given proper arousal, a very large flapdoodle can stretch up to twelve inches or more in length, though most women can manage only seven or eight, and some less than six inches. Depth should not be confused with tightness, however. Even the deepest beaver may have a very tight entrance, since the entrance size is controlled by the pubococcygeal (PC) muscle, a figure eight affair enclosing the anus and vulva. It is this muscle (used by both men and women to control the flow of urine) that involuntarily constricts in a painful female medical condition called vaginismus. During childbirth or after too much sex with an enormous member it can become stretched.

Getting back the old tone involves the woman doing a number of easy exercises, and takes about six weeks:

THE KEGEL EXERCISES FOR WOMEN

First she must establish which is her pubococcygeal, or PC, muscle. This is easy. It is the one she uses to interrupt her urine flow when she goes to the bathroom. To exercise it, she simply imagines that she is having to stop herself peeing.

1. Contract and relax the muscle twenty times.

2. Contract the muscle, hold for three seconds, and then relax. Repeat ten times.

3. Contract the muscle while inhaling. Women should try to avoid contracting their stomach muscles at the same time. This will be difficult at first, but becomes easier with practice. Repeat ten times.

The exercises can of course be done at any time, without anybody knowing.

The woman who does these three or four times a day will quickly see results. "The Kegels were a godsend," wrote one lady. "They really put back the sensations I used to have after I lost my virginity." A Cincinnati schoolteacher added: "About a month ago, during sex, I began contracting my PC muscle, and my partner went crazy and absolutely loved it—at first it was tiring, but after a while it got me even more excited. It's a good tip." It also appears that women with well-toned PC muscles experience more pleasurable, intense orgasms.

The most famous large and tight vagina in literature belongs to one Eskimo Nell, a Wild West woman who is courted by Deadeye Dick, whose "muscular prick" is famous "from the Horn to Panama." The poem, by Anonymous, concerns a coital contest in Black Mike's saloon. I'll spare you the remorseless details and get to the result:

Then she gave a sigh and sucked him dry,
With the ease of a vacuum cleaner . . .

He slipped to the floor and he knew no more,
his passion extinct and dead,
Nor did he shout as his tool came out,
It was stripped right down to a thread.

Only the outer third of the vagina is especially sensitive to touch. The inner two-thirds are so insensitive in some women that certain operations can be performed without anesthetic. Shudder.

Within the vagina is the hymen. This is a curious piece, found only in humans, and quite unlike most people imagine it to be. It's a thin, pliable membrane blocking the entrance of the vagina, but it is hardly ever a complete blockage. When it is, it has to be surgically opened because otherwise the menstrual fluid couldn't come out. In most women the hymen is perforated in some way or another, and often it is not present at all (which is why loss of virginity is painful for some and not for others). This simple, unappreciated biological fact has cost many women their lives. In the Yungar society of Australia, for example, the hymen of a young woman was inspected by two old women a week before her marriage, and ruptured. If no hymen was found, or one that was naturally or sexually perforated to a great degree, the girl was tortured and often murdered. Inserting tampons and some forms of strenuous exercise that put the area under stress may tear the hymen without a penis getting within five miles.

Not only is lack of hymen no proof of sexual activity, presence of hymen is no proof of chastity. Some hymens are so flexible that a woman can have a dozen bouts of intercourse without tearing it. But even then you're not on safe ground. In Japan women sometimes get new hymens using plastic surgery.

During defloration there need not be any blood. If you belong to a community that demands to see the sheets on the day after the wedding, and the face-saving stains are not present, use chicken blood as they do in the Mediterranean.

Something like 70 percent of women report that their first experience of penetrative sex was a painful fiasco, often so that they are put off sex for a long time afterward. Much misery can be avoided if the man proceeds *very slowly,* gives plenty of lead-up stimulation, and ensures that there is adequate lubrication, even if only K-Y jelly: first-night nerves often result in the woman having no natural vaginal secretions at all.

Lubrication

Lubrication can be a source of strife between men and women because for centuries the "dripping cunt" has been crudely symbolic of female sexual arousal. Being wet between the legs does not mean one is necessarily ready for penetration. As I discussed in chapter 2, many factors contribute to a woman feeling that the time is right for hanky-panky. Take it as a demand for immediate penetration and you're likely to get a slap in the face for your impudence. All it means is you are on the right track.

The lubricating fluid is clear, slippery, and slightly scented. It not only lets you slip in and out with ease, but also counteracts the acidity of the canal, which would otherwise do unpleasant things to your semen. Many things can change the degree of vaginal moisture: the pill, tampons, tension, her suddenly wishing you were anywhere except in her bed. However, don't assume that she's not turned on just because she isn't wet. Not only do individuals vary considerably, but any one woman may differ from year to year. Jacinta is thirty-five years old and perfectly healthy:

> I'd always been absolutely normal in that my vagina got pleasantly wet when I was aroused. Then one day for no reason it didn't. I was so worried I actually had tests to see if I was getting an early menopause. I wasn't and

after about four months I returned to normal. The doctor had no explanation for it, and urged me to accept that it didn't matter. Which it didn't.

The lady with the pussy like a geyser who keeps cropping up in pornography is rare in real life—and her wetness is more probably a result of the female equivalent of ejaculation.

When I climax there is a great rush of liquid from my vagina. It isn't slick like my lubrication, but it smells the same. I can't really climax without it. I would be terribly embarrassed to have to explain this to a new sexual partner. I can't for the life of me figure out a way to explain I'm not urinating. I enjoy the sensation greatly . . . I can make it last as long as I want and it often soaks a good part of the bedclothes.

Women have known for centuries that sometimes, at the moment of orgasm, an amount of fluid is ejected. Some men can actually feel it happening high up inside the vagina. A few deaf people persist in insisting it is urine, although it is nothing of the sort. Very similar to the normal vaginal secretions, female ejaculation fluid is colorless, clear, and quite inoffensive. It *may* (the scientific jury is still out on this one) be the feminine equivalent of seminal fluid and *may,* sometimes, be the result of stimulating the G-spot (see p. 190). It has been observed to occur mostly in women with strong pubococcygeal muscles (women with a tight pussy, in common parlance). If vaginal dryness is a problem, K-Y jelly or a special vagina-lubricating gel are available from drugstores. If you've been sent to buy it, don't assume the K-Y is less embarrassing to ask for . . . it's notoriously used by homosexuals for lubricating bottoms. In a tight moment, olive oil would do the trick, as well as allowing you to remark humorously that it says "extra virgin" on the label.

Lack of lubrication is one of the main causes of . . .

Painful Sex

Most women experience pain during sex at some time or another, and it does nothing to add to our affection for men. It can range from the occasional dull throb (quite common) to acute agony. Apart from poor lubrication and uncomfortable settings, the main sources of trouble are:

1. Common medical conditions. Women routinely suffer from at least one of a whole range of conditions such as yeast infection and cystitis. The man's role is to be aware that this is part of a woman's lot (the nature of the vagina makes it prone to infection), and that it does *not* mean the woman has slept with the local football team. It's always awkward if something strikes in the middle of sex and one has to ask the man to withdraw, so please be considerate: don't sulk, and don't imply she's making a fuss over nothing (some of these conditions are very painful).

2. Uncommon medical conditions, such as a radical hysterectomy, can cause pain inside. Vaginismus affects 2–3 percent of adult women—it is a condition whereby the vaginal muscles contract painfully and make penetration (or, more awkwardly, withdrawal) impossible. Advice to men as in case 1, only more so.

3. Certain positions in which there is very deep penetration, particularly where the woman is lying on her back with her legs up, or intercourse from behind. In any position, excessive vigorous pumping can also cause acute pain because eventually one thrust will go too far.

4. Outsized penis. A point to boost the morale of men with small ones: "Why do men want big ones? They *hurt*!" Even when a large penis enters a large woman a certain amount of caution should be observed. Make sure she is *fully* aroused before penetration, and go slowly.

5. Going on too long. The pain may be because her position has become uncomfortable, or because the lubrication has dried up. If you suspect either, offer to bring things to a close. One can usually sense if one's partner has lost interest when they no longer respond so enthusiastically with the "mmmm's" and "aaahhhh's".

6. Others: "It's bad if I am being 'stabbed' at, or if a piece of outside skin from my lips gets pinched in somehow or hair is pulled." Constipation can cause pain, because the rectal canal runs right alongside the vaginal one.

If intercourse is consistently painful a woman should see a doctor.

How Many Positions for Penetration Are There?

As many as you care to imagine. *The Perfumed Garden,* written by Sheikh Nefzaoui in the sixteenth century, lists thirty-six. Of these, twenty-five "can only be practiced if both man and woman are free from physical defects, and of analogous construction; for instance, one or the other of them must not be humpbacked." More recently, a German gym teacher, with admirable Teutonic thoroughness, calculated mathematically that there were 531 distinct, reasonable positions.

Actually, it is not the Eastern erotic books that recommend idiotic positions so much as the erotic art, particularly when it appears on a holy temple. Ripping the woman's tendons at the groin and cracking her spine in an effort to satisfy one man orally and another genitally are particular favorites of the religiously minded. Another curious tactic involves suspending the woman in a harness, bottom parts nethermost, and getting a servant to lower her onto the awaiting organ.

I, like many women, find this particular subject vastly overrated. Most peculiar sexual positions are uncomfortable and lousy for orgasm. Therefore, make sure you know the answer to . . .

Which Position Does Your Partner Prefer?

It's likely to be the missionary, which is very popular with women. With a new partner, go for this one until instructed otherwise.

Getting the right position is one of the most important aspects of enjoyable sex for women, and if you launch into something requiring double joints and builder's scaffolding the result is likely to be a disaster. Fancy work is better left until you know each other well (extremely well, in some cases). For purposes of satisfaction we prefer the old familiars. Even apart from comfort there is another very good reason for this: men get aroused by novel approaches, while women usually get distracted. The first illustrated edition of the *Kama Sutra* was a sad day for women across the whole country:

Mr. Pottle: First we put your leg here, on the mantel. No, the right leg. Then this one crosses over and touches your ear. Now touch your elbow with your nose while I slip my left foot under your chin—don't be theatrical, I just washed it—and put my other leg, where? But that's ridiculous. I'm really enjoying this, aren't you? Who made that noise? Not me. I wonder if the Bennets do this. I'll bet they don't.

Mrs. Pottle: Are you sure it won't hurt your hemorrhoids, dear?

Mr. P.: Ah, there, got it, now, oo . . .

Mrs. P.: Well?

Mr. P.: Oh dear.

Mrs. P.: Oh dear! Already!

Mr. P.: Um, ah, 'fraid so, let me, um, get you a tissue.

"The main reason I stopped having sex with Michael," complained Julia, nineteen, "was because he did everything under the sun but the obvious one. I felt I had no contact with him. He said he worshipped my body and that's why he wanted to do all this, but really he worshipped something completely impersonal. I wasn't Julia anymore, I was that girl with the big boobs and supple tendons."

Don't worry about seeming unadventurous. As with most exotic sexual practices, if women want them it's far easier in today's climate to suggest the wild stuff than it is the tame. The hardest thing is when a girl is simply longing for good old-fashioned sex and the boyfriend cajoles her instead into bending backward over the kitchen stove.

Of course fancy positions are often sexy as an oddity. But the oddity value wears off quickly. If variability is what's lacking in your relationship, it's a much better bet to vary the places you have sex, and the times, and the surrounding circumstances than the position itself. Women are most likely to cite these occasions as pleasantly memorable.

I was once helping my boyfriend fix his car, which was standing just outside his garage, in front of a row of houses. It was a green sports car, very racy, and all of a sudden he pulled me into the garage and slid down the garage door. We fucked standing up, leaning over the car hood—and thinking of all those neighbors' eyes outside. It was incredibly uncomfortable, but very very sexy.

Man on Top

The good old missionary gets abused for a whole host of reasons. It's "boring" and "obvious." It's "old-fashioned," because everybody knows it has something to do with Victorian Bible-bashers and natives in reed huts. It's "politically incorrect," because the man's position shows he's a male chauvinist pig whose sole object in life is to oppress a woman.

Don't believe a word of it. The missionary is position number one and I think it deserves a more glamorous name. Suggestions to be submitted on a postcard—a Mars Bar and a signed copy of *How to Have an Orgasm* for the best. It's extremely comfortable, provided you're not lying on the concrete floor of the garage with an overweight man, and it gives reasonably good clitoral stimulation. Exhaustive studies of tribes and cultures the world over reveal that it is the most popular sexual position there is. The only people who don't like it are the Trobriand islanders, who consider the white man a "slob who is through much too quickly. He crushes his poor wife. He lies so heavily on her that she cannot participate properly." As a poor Western woman who has been often so crushed, let me add that I find the experience very pleasant.

Other advantages to bear in mind: you can kiss and do peculiar things with ears and necks. It allows you to gaze into each other's eyes *or* to face away and *not* look at each other.

I like the missionary best because I can hold on and forget. I like to feel his weight on top of me and his hips between my thighs. When Mack does it, he's great. He begins slowly. Eases his penis in. Sometimes he doesn't go all the way at first. He plays around with the head of his penis just inside where I'm the most sensitive. After a bit I want him all, so I can feel him all over and get the pressure between my legs. I don't like a lot of thrusting. It doesn't do much for me on its own. It's better when he moves slowly. He can stay still and let me move my own hips. That's the rule: begin slowly and then get slower. When I get excited I lift my legs up and circle his waist. I love coming like that, gripping him inside.

There's one disadvantage that I can think of: getting my hand in. I come only if I use my hand too. But with him on top it's not as easy. I can get there and masturbate myself even when he presses down. It's sexy. It's if I think this man disapproves of that or feels it's a slur on his ability, then it's the worst position to try and explain away why you're doing it.

Many women also like this position because being covered by a man minimizes all their worries about flab, stretch marks, bosom shape, etc., all of which should never be underestimated in their power to spoil sex.

There are a number of adjustments to the basic missionary position that help to provide extra clitoral stimulation:

It depends on what you need and with some couples where the clitoris is in relation to his pressure parts. To get it right he might have to prop himself on his elbows or I put my legs between his instead of the other way. A man can easily tell when he's got there on me. There's an immediate increase in the number of "Um-mmmms." My body gets tenser. I spread my legs more to get as much of him as possible.

Another very important trick: get your partner to clasp your but-tocks and control your movements in and out in the way that best suits her. That way you'll get a good idea of what she wants most without having the awkwardness of asking.

People say missionary doesn't give women enough control. Yes it does! She uses her hands to dictate the pace. He knows he can stop and rest if he's about to ejaculate. I've gone to sleep with Nigel in this position and we've woken up refreshed and had another twenty minutes. When he gets too close, he stops or pulls out. He knows I'm not going to make a sudden movement that will tip him over into climax. Better still, I know it too. With control, it's easily the best.

Woman on Top

This second most popular position was once thought risqué: a certain indication that the woman was morally corrupt and the man either depraved or spineless. It is now considered de rigueur in all Hollywood sex scenes (especially those starring Greta Scacchi).

Notably, societies that believe a woman's satisfaction is vital to good sex are fond of this position. It gives the woman plenty of control. She can dictate the degree of penetration, the speed, and the rhythm much better than when she's down below, and it also allows clitoral stimulation, "though it's hard on the hand," says Graham. "You got to kind of twist. My wife likes me to use my thumb. Put it just above my private part and she can use it. I keep still." This position also lessens the feeling some women have of being subservient to the man.

I don't know why, the idea of "sitting" on a man turns me on. I want to sit on his lap, sit on his face, sit on his penis . . . he's passive and underneath me. Liam says to me: "Sit on me, sit on me." I clutch him inside and keep moving while I have an orgasm. Because I get really wet at orgasm and when he ejaculates it all flows out again, there's wet everywhere. I keep humping him because the warm liquid is so nice. He's young. He can take it!

Although this extra control leads sex therapists to recommend it as the best position for women who have difficulty climaxing, the point can be overdone. Sitting upright she is in full glare, and many women feel *extremely* self-conscious not only about their breasts (she could wear a T-shirt) but about their facial expressions. "I know it sounds silly, but I am so embarrassed when Mark looks at my face when I'm aroused. I feel exposed, and I can't relax enough to climax."

In his book *Super Potency: A Doctor's Guide to Better Sex — At Any Age,* the unpromisingly named Dr. E. Flatto recommends this position as best for men who want to control their ejaculation. Hhhmmmmm. In my experience men find the sight of the woman on top having her way with them too sexy for good self-control.

Side to Side

Favored by the Masai and recommended by Ovid, Roman author of *The Art of Love,* "side to side" is an umbrella term for all manner of peculiarities, many of which are hardly side to side at all, but back to side and side to back. It can be clumsy, but, when done correctly, it is a calm position because neither partner can move too rapidly. It's bad for clitoral stimulation, unless you're wedged in a narrow gap between two walls. Joyce writes, after completing a round-the-world trip:

Good for Indian trains! They'd overpacked the train, so my boyfriend had to sleep on the same single bunk as me, and there wasn't any curtain either. We lay side by side being lulled to sleep by the movement of the train and the hot night. Sometimes the train would stop for a long time in the middle of nowhere and I could hear the crickets and the guards. At one point I put my hand down to scratch my leg and felt Tom's penis bunched up beneath his cotton pants. So I lifted my skirt and moved myself against this mound (pretending to be asleep as well, of course!) and rubbed my panties against him in time with the train. I think I came. I don't remember. When I woke up a second time he'd pulled my panties off and was fucking me. I had to hold his mouth to stop him making so much noise. When he ejaculated he almost threw me out of the bed it was so extreme.

According to the ancient Chinese health manual *Goddess of the Shell,* a man should penetrate a woman twice a day, eighteen strokes each, for fifteen consecutive days, in this position, if he wants to concentrate his semen.

The Starfish

The most underrated position of them all. It sounds hideously complicated to describe in words, but is actually very easy to get into. Your partner lies on her back. You lie to her right, resting on your left side. She now lifts her right leg up, enabling you to slot your right leg beneath it and over the top of her left leg. Your right thigh now lies between her legs, enabling you to slip your penis into her. You can maneuver your torsos reasonably distant from each other, or close enough to kiss. Adjust to suit.

The Starfish is one of the greats. In his book *Oragenitalism,* G. Legman (who, along with Semans, Lopiccolo, and Heiman, joins a long list of aptly named sex book writers) calls it the scissors, the horizontal cross, or the T-upside-down. It is "probably the best of all coital postures," he says, and then devotes five pages to explaining why, the chief reason being that it is a good way to progress from oral sex to intercourse without the cumbersome clambering around that the other positions require. I leave it up to you to see if you agree.

The Starfish has a host of advantages for women. It is, first,

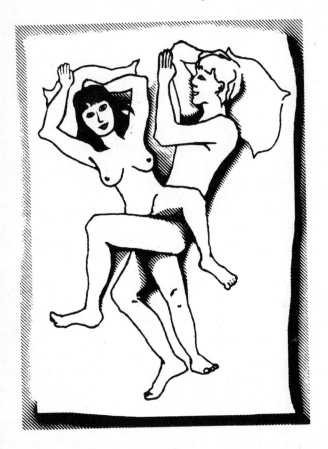

The Starfish

very comfortable. Neither of you has to support the other and it's open to so many slight variations that it can be adjusted to suit all figures and heights, and you don't get a sore back or pins and needles when sex goes on for a long time. It is also a private position. There are times—speaking as a woman—when you want to look your lover in the face, and times when you need to be left alone to concentrate:

> I always want to be near Fred. I adore looking at him. He's my dream. But if I want to enjoy sex fully, I have to concentrate or, more to the point, not feel that I'm being concentrated on. Kissing and the rest. I want it before and after, but when I'm really feeling sexy, I have to focus my mind on the sex. Besides, if we need to touch and kiss, we can still do it.

> Yes, you're right, "Starfish" is great! Jonathan is not very handsome, so I can cover him up with the bedspread and think about someone else.

The Starfish allows the woman easy access to her own parts. She can rub herself without trouble, even without the man knowing; she can position his leg over her pubis and across her stomach so that it presses in a satisfying manner. If he's drunk or too sleepy to know what he's doing, the Starfish enables the woman to keep going without difficulty. And it's marvelous for morning sex, when all a person wants is the essentials, not the sight and smell of a groggy partner.

The Chinese health manual also has something to say about what appears to be the Starfish position, more or less: to strengthen the man's bones, forty-five thrusts, five times a day, for ten days; to increase his blood circulation, fifty-four thrusts, six times a day, for twenty days.

This is some fit Chinaman.

Sitting Down

This is the least-used position, because it takes a lot of energy, is usually uncomfortable, and movement is restricted. One version of it—when the man squats in front of the woman who is lying down, and she straddles his thighs with her legs—is popular with tribes the world over, and was in fact the position that so shocked the missionaries into insisting upon the missionary. In this position all stimulation for the woman is manual at this stage, but as things progress the man may pull her up so that they are both in a semierect squatting or kneeling position. Altogether very hard work, best left to those who have done it since childhood to the tune of Pacific waves beneath the coconut trees. For the unpracticed it's best to

> both sit in a chair that is low enough for the woman to touch her feet on the ground behind so that she can rotate her hips and push up and down. I caught one of my boyfriends with his bare legs slipped underneath the arms of a chair, playing with himself, which is how I learned about it. He liked the idea of being "locked in" I suppose. I expect his mom had kept him in a closet. But he'd forgotten to lock the bedroom door. He was still mumbling excuses as I got myself onto his lap, facing him, which was quite easy to do because it was a low chair with high arms, like the type Viking kings sit in, quaffing from goblets and reciting sagas. As I rose up and down, he licked my breasts and sucked them like a baby. Seventh heaven!

The ease and quality of standing penetration depends on the relative sizes of the two partners. Ideally, the woman should be slightly longer in the legs than the man, and then (to make up for it) slightly shorter in the torso. Or she should be Edith Piaf sized, to be lifted as if putting on a backpack the wrong way around. Shower (and bath) intercourse is dangerous, slippery, and uncomfortable. Don't use soap and beware of the fittings. Jayne was off work for three weeks because her boyfriend let go of her at the crucial moment and the tap went into her right buttock.

Man Enters from Behind

If mutual oral sex is 69, then this position is 99. "Doggy style," in bar parlance. Penetration from behind is the favorite approach of most four-limbed animals, although orangutans and chimps have been caught doing it in the missionary position, and Aristotle (mistakenly, though for obvious reasons) thought that hedgehogs also do it belly to belly. The *Kama Sutra* mentions ten types of this one form of embrace, each characterized by an animal that the shameless lovers are supposed to imitate while enjoying each other, viz., cow, dog, goat, deer, ass, cat, tiger, elephant, boar, horse.

Ninety-nine is good for quick relief (for him at least) in awkward places, such as in the woods, or behind the rhododendron bush at a garden party. I wouldn't expect to have an orgasm in this position without extra manual stimulation, but the convenience of it makes it ideal for derring-do. The fondest coital memories of some of the women I've spoken to concern sitting on their beloved in a public place when wearing a disguising skirt, and executing a few deft wriggles. Onlookers assume she is doing no more than bouncing playfully on the man's lap. Alice, a forty-three-year-old accountant, remarks, "It is incredibly sexy to feel an organ uncontrollably satisfying itself inside you while you're fully dressed in the midst of a busy party (lights down low) and chatting politely to anyone around you":

> I do it quite often this way because I like the feeling of being used. The thought of the man getting his pleasure

from me, like I was just to be thrown away, is some-times very sexy. He just slots me on his penis and fucks me for his own satisfaction. It is uncomplicated and coarse. He grips me around the waist and when he comes he falls down on top of me. I imagine being made to do it under a table, kneeling between two men neither knowing what the other is up to, so that they have to keep a serious conversation going while they jerk off inside me. I'm quite ashamed of myself for thinking about this so often.

Paradoxically, one of the most popular aspects of 99 is that it takes the pressure off women to have to climax. Since the man is behind, on the opposite side of the woman's clitoris, the sex is uncomplicated by concerns about getting enough time for her own orgasm or his disappointment/accusations when she doesn't come. It becomes pure sex.

Man Enters up the Behind

She returns and anoints him thoroughly (with Vaseline), with an icy expert touch. Harry shudders. Thelma lies down beside him with her back turned, curls forward as if to be shot from a cannon, and reaches behind to guide him. "Gently."

It seems it won't go, but suddenly it does. The medicinal odor of displaced Vaseline reaches his nostrils. The grip is tight at the base, but beyond, whereas cunt is all velvety suction and caress, there is no sensation: a void, a pure black box, a casket of perfect nothingness. He is in that void, past her tight ring of muscle.

—John Updike, *Rabbit Is Rich*

I've watched a lot of porno films and every single one has concentrated upon anal sex. (I remember once a blond Swede was
on all fours with her head in the washing machine.) From this
I must conclude that doing it up women's bottoms is a top male
fantasy.

Women are more cautious. Anal sex can be horribly painful
and extremely dangerous. It is the easiest way to catch AIDS
and a host of other sexually transmitted diseases, because the
rectal tissues are much more delicate than the vaginal ones and
easily lacerated. All the same, it is a more popular activity than
people imagine.

One in ten American heterosexual couples have anal sex
regularly, and up to half have tried it once or twice; the UK is
probably not far behind these figures. It is particularly common
in African and Latin cultures, where contraceptives are hard to
come by and where virginity in brides is valued. In a survey of
5,514 Canadian college students, one in five of the women had
had anal intercourse. A similar study in Puerto Rico came up
with a figure of one in three. In other words,

---

*MANY MORE HETEROSEXUALS ENGAGE IN SODOMY
THAN HOMOSEXUALS.*

"The traditional and continuing medical and scientific silence
about heterosexual anal intercourse is so deafening that it begs
to be noticed," wrote Dr. Bruce Voeller in a recent forty-page
academic paper entitled "AIDS and Heterosexual Anal Intercourse." It is a major factor in the spread of AIDS.

Women don't enjoy the same pleasure from anal sex as
male homosexuals do, because we don't have a prostate gland,
which can be pleasantly stimulated by this activity. For women,
it is rarely comfortable and must be done *only with full, un-*

pressured consent, and then very, very gradually. The chief attraction is that the idea is sexy and the act extremely intimate. Done from the front, it allows clitoral stimulation. The following responses are typical of women's widely divergent opinions about anal sex. You might hit lucky with your partner, but don't be surprised if you're regarded as a pervert.

> I do it now and again, but only with a man I know very well and feel very close to. It's too important. It's the greatest violation. A man who does that to you has done everything possible. There's nothing secret left.

> I think the idea is revolting. I'd never let my husband do it to me. I'd be disgusted if he even suggested it.

> It is a very odd feeling, especially afterwards. To begin with it can be agony, and then inside he has to move very slowly. But after it's come out it's unsettling, like you have to go to the bathroom but can't.

Mary is the only woman who described a fantasy of anal sex:

> I am a young girl in a Victorian seminary. Although we are teenagers, we of course know nothing about sex: absolutely nothing. The head of the school is a man. When we are naughty he devises this punishment: we must lift our skirts and petticoats, and bend over. Of course, we understand that naughty children get their bottoms smacked, even though we are fourteen years old.
>
> We feel the punishment on our bottoms. What we don't know is that the head has unbuttoned his trousers, taken out his prick and is having complete liberty with us. Sometimes he pushes it between the cheeks of our bottoms. Sometimes he penetrates our bottoms. He keeps his highly respectable school going for twenty years. The girls grow up very disciplined.

The only way to find out if your partner is interested in anal sex is to ask her—accidentally on purpose arriving in the wrong orifice is cowardly and low. If she agrees, use a sterile lubricant like K-Y jelly (the rectum produces no lubricant of its own) and a strong condom if you have any doubts about your health or the health of your previous partners. Note, however, that Vaseline and other petroleum-based products should *not* be used because they degrade the latex of the condom. K-Y jelly is okay. Withdraw carefully afterward and don't touch the woman's vaginal area at all until you've washed thoroughly, or you will give her a nasty infection. Similarly, *never* move from anal to vaginal penetration without a thorough wash *and* change of condom, otherwise sex is likely to be off the menu for several weeks.

For logophiles: the word sodomy comes from Sodom, the city on the plains of Jordan that was destroyed by the Lord for being a den of iniquity. In fact, the Bible never specifies what the naughty Sodomites got up to. It doesn't even state whether it was sexual or not. The city's sin might have been anything from excessive pride to transvestism to cannibalism. It was only in the first century A.D. that the church decreed that the Sodomites had been buggering each other, largely because that is what those enemies of the church, the Greeks and Romans, did.

Buggery is another odd word. It comes from "Bulgari," the medieval name for Bulgarian, and refers to the heretics who lived there. One sect advocated abstaining from procreation (rather a self-defeating tactic) and the term came to refer to any sexual deviation from the accepted Christian line. A few etymological steps later it was limited entirely to anal sex.

How to Make Sure You Enter the Correct Orifice

A serious consideration. The practiced man will usually know what he's about (although mistakes occur even with the experts), but the novice may (and should) be worried. Women have three orifices down there (although only two are penetrable) and the terrain is as confusing as the Grand Canyon. Things are particularly liable to go wrong when penetrating from behind. Many a girl has been lying on her tummy sweetly waiting for vaginal intercourse, only to be rudely awakened by a taut, probing penis on its way into her bottom.

The simple solution is to let the woman guide you with her hand. There's nothing in the least shaming in suggesting she does this. If she offers no guidance, then proceed as follows.

Woman lying on her back: Rest the length of your penis between her legs and against her mons (the part with pubic hair), then move the penis tip down, nudging gently until it is able to penetrate. The part you're after is this side of the halfway mark. Keep it very well lubricated to make the passage easy and obvious.

Woman lying on her front: This time begin by resting your penis between her legs and against the bed, and proceed upward. If you begin by resting your penis against her bottom and moving downward, the first orifice will be her anus.

Ridiculous Things Women Worry about during Intercourse

> I don't feel self-conscious (apart from premenstrually when I feel like a whale) and I'm happy about the lights on, covers off. But I do feel self-conscious in another way. I don't like Gabriel watching my face as I writhe around in ecstasy and I feel embarrassed when I moan or groan when he's making me come . . . Being told that you asked, "Fill me up, big boy—bang inside me," etc., puts you off a little.

Forget about swollen nipples and sex flush, saying horribly embarrassing things is the only infallible mark of satisfaction during sex. They tend to be just the sort of comments you find in the filthiest of filthy literature, which is disconcerting for both of you, especially when your partner is usually a perfect specimen of demure womanhood. Comments about filling, ramming, gushing are particularly popular from women and it is regarded as singular bad taste to remind us of them afterward when normal sense has returned. Not that this is the prerogative of our sex, of course. There's a man I know whose immediate postcoital screech is invariably, "I didn't say it! I didn't say anything!"

"What was that about being milked?" asks his wife, who does not play fair in these matters.

"I don't know what you mean."

"Squeeze me, milk me?"

"Please! I'm trying to sleep. I have to work tomorrow."

"Squeeze me, milk me, *pasteurize* me?"

The following morning he is innocently sitting at breakfast with the paper, when she pushes a bottle across the table. "Pasteurized milk on your cornflakes, darling?"

"I almost got my first boyfriend thrown into an asylum," writes Mrs. Hanson. "What he said was so disgusting I thought he was a deviant. In the day he was the opposite. I thought he was a split personality—a psychopath. I wrote an anonymous letter to the mental home and ran away for a month while they sorted it out."

Next to comments, it's facial expressions. "Will my face contort and look ugly if I let go?" "I must look so unattractive going oooh aaahhh." Women spend their whole *lives* worrying about the way they look, and they're not about to stop just because the curtains are drawn. It's not only expressions. Robbie was over the moon when he successfully lured a red-haired beauty back to his apartment. "I couldn't take my eyes off her, thinking how gorgeous she was, what a lovely complexion and hair, etc. But when we got into bed and I scooped her into my arms, she said, 'Don't kiss me, you'll smudge my makeup.'" Although few women nowadays go to bed in full war paint and hairspray, there are legions of us who hold on doggedly to mascara (which occasionally smudges). A good 50 percent of my toilet-going expeditions are really to check that I don't look like a panda.

Looks, smells, and sounds can spring unpleasant surprises. In the middle of intercourse you may hear peculiar noises from down there, "almost farty noises" as one woman put it. Another explained, "I seem to produce a lot of bubbling and what seems to be excess air from my vagina—not my bottom!" It *is* excess air, very common and only worth a mutual giggle, not awkwardness.

There are scores more things on women's minds: "Should I have shaved my legs?" "Is my vagina tight enough for him?" "I have a slight incontinence problem due to childbirth." "I'm not experienced enough for him." "My red and angry operation scars." It's a most unusual woman who beds a new partner without at least one worry, but sometimes it can get a little out of hand:

> I think about a lot of things during sex . . . "Perhaps I shouldn't be having sex with this guy," "I hate how his breath smells like beer and his clothes smell like cigarettes from living in the bar," "Why am I sleeping with somebody who doesn't love me?" "Why can't I say 'no' to sex?" etc., etc., etc. "What am I going to do if I get pregnant?" "Why is it taking him so long to come?" "Does he like the way that I am doing this?" "Is he tired of kissing my cunt?" "What do I do now—would he like to change positions?" "Is he comfortable?" etc. etc. etc.

> I feel that I get more aroused with my clothes on sometimes because the fear of pregnancy and sexually transmitted diseases really gets to me a lot. So I would say that fears that come creeping in during sex prevent me from getting to orgasm.

Such thoughts seem funny, but they cause a great deal of anguish. Women are more easily distracted during sex than men, and they need all the circumstances to be right before they can enjoy it. If your partner voices her worry don't pooh-pooh it, but think of a realistic reason why she should stop worrying: your answer could be the difference between sexual tension and blissful satisfaction. Here's one I doubt you've come across before:

> I'm afraid he's going to die. My grandfather and father both died when they were having sex. I know he's going to do it too, and then I'll be stuck and won't be able to get out and will have to call the police. Help. Please advise.

When Are Women Most Likely to Be in the Mood?

Human, ape, and monkey females are the only animals in the kingdom that aren't estrous—i.e., they don't have to be in heat to have sex. This is marvelous for everybody. It means we can and do do it every hour of the year, for three-quarters of our lives. However, many women report distinct variations in their desire according to what part of the menstrual cycle they're in. This mysterious affair, with its furtive range of cottony things, TV ads showing pads soaked in *blue* ink, and white swing-top trash cans, lasts—or should last—twenty-eight days, one lunar month. In some women it is naturally irregular, but menstruation can also be disrupted by contraceptives, dieting, stress, and, as every anxious adulterer knows, pregnancy.

A small proportion of women notice no variation in sexual desire over the whole four weeks; the remainder divide in two ways. Less than half say they feel a definite upsurge in sexiness midway between two periods, during ovulation. This is the time when women are most fertile, so check your contraceptives.

The rest slightly favor the days leading up to a period—days twenty-five to twenty-eight. If you and your girlfriend are living miles apart, or if you're in one of those peculiar prisons that allows "family" visits every month, choose the day of your privileges with care.

However, to ensure nothing is too easy, nature ordains that for some of us the week before a period is by far and away the *least* sexy time of month. Water retention makes women feel puffy and bloated, breasts are tender, and premenstrual syndrome (PMS) causes frustration, anger, or depression. Queen Victoria suffered from PMS so severely that "even [Lord] Melbourne, a past master at dealing with women, had on one occasion quavered and feared to sit down as the fire blazed in the eyes of the eighteen-year-old queen." There are several cases in which a woman tormented with extreme PMS has actually killed. So approach with caution. Don't pick days twenty-five to twenty-eight to start complaining about the bills.

Most of us are less harassed. Barbara, thirty-eight, becomes simply peculiar: "My body and my emotions fill up and slow down. I get obsessed with licorice pieces. If my husband wants me, he hides some and bribes me later, but it doesn't do him much good. I usually snatch them and tell him to piss off. My little sister is the opposite. It affects her positively. She's always picking up men then. She can't get enough. My big sister gets depressed, knocks off work, and sits in front of the TV all day griping. Nothing is right."

If men menstruated they would be surprised at the degree of pain that regularly goes with it. When I was twenty-two, after several years of quite simple periods, I began getting such terrible cramps that for two or three days each month I would be writhing and crying with the pain. This lasted ten years, and then got better. Most women suffer at least discomfort for a few days, either in their pelvis or their breasts. All such responses are tied up with women's complex hormonal system and *not figments of the imagination*.

Can I Make Love to a Woman Who Is Menstruating?

Of course you can.

Providing she is willing, there is no earthly reason to desist. A lot of women find the idea extremely erotic, others will think you're a pervert. It's a bit mucky if her periods are heavy, but this can be avoided if (in addition to her usual contraceptive) she asks the doctor to fit her with a contraceptive diaphragm. This is a thick rubber dome attached to a flexible ring that fits inside the vagina, high up against her cervix. It can be removed when not needed and stored in a thing that looks similar to a powder compact. The diaphragm's usual purpose is, of course, to block sperm from reaching the danger zone, but it can just as easily work in the opposite direction for a short time. She should be careful to remove it over the toilet bowl or in a bathtub as there will be a gush of blood.

Some men find the whole business extremely sexy:

> I had one lover who was really turned on by menstrual blood; he could tell by smelling me that I had my period, and couldn't wait to give me oral sex. There was something very liberating about his desire for me during what I had always thought of as an undesirable time. Having said that, I have never met a man who was unwilling to make love to me during my period.

Another woman found a novel cure for menstrual pains. "Sex becomes really uncomfortable if the blood flow has been heavy with cramping. However, oral sex seems to ease the cramping."

And, just for the record, I vigorously support the use of the term the Curse to describe women's menstruation. Far from "denying our womanhood" (as overzealous politically correct people have it), the Curse is an affectionate, lighthearted name.

Also I would not deny schoolgirls the pleasure of their stifled giggles when the English teacher solemnly reads aloud from Tennyson's "The Lady of Shalott":

> Out flew the web and floated wide;
> The mirror crack'd from side to side;
> "The curse has come upon me," cried the Lady of Shalott.

Contraception

WITH ALL THE
pills,
IUDs,
condoms,
diaphragms,
safe periods,
coitus interruptus,
abortions,
accidents,
wars,
and emigration,

why is the bus so crowded?
—ZYGMUNT FRANKEL

Penetration almost always means contraception. And, despite a host of modern methods, *contraception is a difficult business for women*. Men nowadays might be forgiven for believing that we're spoiled for choice and that the whole subject is wonderfully easy. It isn't. Unless a woman is very lucky, finding something safe, painless, and reliable is a great nuisance.

First the magic **pill.** Imagine how you would feel each

morning if, on waking, you reached for your contraceptive pill and read: *Warning: this pill may cause depression, thrombosis, heart disease, hypertension, and weight gain.* (Lately the warnings have gotten sterner still.) Up to 40 percent of women suffer some kind of very unpleasant side effect, including fatal blood clotting. I tried the pill, got hugely fat, extremely depressed, and eventually went off sex altogether (thus obviating the need for contraception in the first place). Mine was a common response. The pill also makes the vagina more susceptible to fungal infections that rule out sex. Even supposing a woman suffers no immediate side effects, it's not infallible. If she forgets a day, or suffers vomiting or diarrhea before the contraceptive components have time to be absorbed, she can fall pregnant. On the other hand, if all goes well, the pill (which is the collective term for all oral contraceptives) has a less than one percent failure rate.

Then there is the **diaphragm.** I had one of these too. Nasty, rubbery things that have to be first fitted by a doctor (my friend's doctor set her up with the wrong size and so she got pregnant: doctor's mistake, her burden for the rest of her life). Each time a woman has sex the damn thing must be carefully inserted and filled with spermicide (thus ruling out oral sex for her). They are messy, awkward, and ruin spontaneous sex. The rubber gets smelly fairly soon. Diaphragms have the advantage that there are no serious side effects, though some people are allergic to the latex of the diaphragm or to certain types of spermicide. The failure rate is 3 percent: not high on the face of it, but alarming if you use the diaphragm for years and years.

Interestingly, diaphragms filled with spermicide are one of the oldest contraceptive devices. The approach is to use a physical barrier together with something acidic because the acid kills the sperm. Sponges soaked in vinegar were used even in Christ's time, while the ancient Egyptians employed tips of the acacia tree combined with lint and honey. Casanova, before he set to work, would gallantly insert into his ladies a hollowed-out lemon.

The **intrauterine device** (**IUD**) or **coil** has to be professionally fitted, which can be extremely painful if one's innards decide to go into spasm. If this happens the coil is usually impossible to fit at all. A successful insertion means the coil remains way up out of reach of fingers or penises, with only a small loop hanging down for eventual removal, for up to five years. This, of course, gives the wearer blissful freedom and I am a great supporter of the coil. However, because it carries an increased risk of infections that can lead to infertility, it is not commonly prescribed for women who have not completed their family. Further disadvantages are bad period pains, heavier blood flow, and the possibility that one's body will become temperamental and spontaneously reject this "foreign object," sometimes without the wearer herself knowing (result: pregnancy). Strangely, though putting something into the uterus for contraception has a venerable history (Arabs have put round stones in the uteri of their camels for centuries), no one to this day knows how the IUD works.

A **male pill**? Questionable. What will the health risks be and how long will it take to discover them? Can a woman trust a one-night stand who says he's on the male pill, when (if ever) it eventually arrives on the market? I couldn't feel comfortable about sex unless I'd actually seen him swallow the thing every day that month.

Sterilization is the serious option, especially for men. Do this and a woman's worries about you are over, although it must be your decision, not hers. The operation is very simple and can be performed under local anesthetic in fifteen minutes (one doctor actually did it to himself). Afterward a man can get an erection and ejaculate just as before, except that there's a little less semen, because the part containing the sperm is missing. The operation is intended to be permanent, but you have an approximately 50 percent chance of successful reversal (the longer you leave it the worse are your chances).

Female sterilization is a much more complicated operation, and the chances for reversal are practically zero.

Don't rely on the **rhythm method.** Its basic approach assumes that a woman's menstrual cycle is always regular (it isn't) and that her fertility within the cycle varies according to a set pattern (it doesn't). Other approaches depend on variations in body temperature and changes in cervical mucus, and they're all useless. One might just as well use the old methods of jumping backward, sneezing, and telling jokes.

As for the **withdrawal method,** don't even give it a serious thought. It's considerably worse than the rhythm method because it messes up sex as well. The man must withdraw his penis in the nick of time, just before he ejaculates. This not only takes extraordinary self-control, but meanwhile the woman is gnashing her teeth in fear that the event will be mistimed or overlooked. Even if you succeed you must then hope and pray that no rogue sperm have sneaked out prior to ejaculation (they often do). If you mistime, and the semen spills inside the woman, there are **douches.** You've got thirty seconds to kill 900 million spermatozoa before they make it into the safety of the cervix.

In regard to contraception we are still, writes Alan Guttmacher, one of the pioneers in the field, in the "horse and buggy days" of effective measures.

I hope that understanding the difficulties that women face with regard to contraception will make men more flexible in agreeing to their partner's suggestions. If she asks you to wear a condom, don't make her task even more difficult by comments along the lines of "It's like having a bath with your socks on." Younger women, studies have shown, are particularly susceptible to pressure from their boyfriends, which is one reason why the teenage pregnancy statistics are so dreadful.

A responsible attitude to birth control significantly enhances a man's attractiveness, and makes him seem decent and mature. Even the most super-sophisticated lover drops to rock bottom if he's unhelpful in this department. In the heat of desire it's easy to forget that it's her body that will carry the mistake for nine months, and that the baby will be her responsibility for life. If she can prove paternity you will be liable to contribute to its upkeep.

And finally, it's not in the least "presumptuous" for either sex to carry their own condoms, just highly sensible.

Impotence

Every man suffers from impotence occasionally. Most of the time it's nothing more than the result of too much pressure at work, anxiety about sexual performance, or too little sleep. As long as your concern doesn't get out of hand, it cures itself in a couple of nights.

Long-term impotence affects one in every seven men, becoming increasingly probable with age. A quarter of men are impotent by the time they're sixty. Ten years later, 60 percent have difficulty getting an erection. At eighty, only 15 percent of men do not suffer from impotence although at least half are still interested in sex. Chronic impotence that is not age-related is extremely common and usually puts the sadness of Job into the sufferer, yet in most cases it is simple to cure.

There are, broadly speaking, two types of impotence: the type due to psychological causes, and that due to physical ones. Until very recently, the medical profession followed Freud (who was himself impotent for much of his life) and assumed that nine out of ten cases were psychological. Now it's known that most impotence is actually due to physical causes—any illness from the most mild upward may bring it on, because the body, when it has to spend a large amount of energy on restoring health, is inclined to consider sexual activity a luxury. King Louis XVI of France could not get an erection until he was twenty-three because his foreskin was too tight.

Because a few illnesses (diabetes, for example) have well-established links with impotence, any extended loss of potency should send you to the doctor. But physically caused impotence may be due to something that can be easily dealt with, such as a bad diet. Hamburger, fries, and Coke for breakfast, lunch, and dinner will do neither the waistline nor the old pecker any good at all. Smoking clogs up the arteries, making it hard for blood to get into the penis. Cut down on cigarettes, switch to low-sugar, low-salt products, and ensure that every day you eat a good quantity of raw, fresh fruit and vegetables.

More and more serious attention is given nowadays to diet and its effects on our health. Constipation, for example, which is almost always due to eating too little fiber, is cited by Dr. Flatto, in his book *Super Potency,* as a major "potency killer." Exercise is also extremely important for sexual health. If a man wants to remain potent for his whole life, the best thing he can do is concentrate on being generally fit. A little bit of walking or swimming every day will soon do a considerable amount of good. In a study conducted with sedentary but healthy men, published in the *Archives of Sexual Behaviour,* the authors found that exercise and reduced fat consumption allows increased blood flow, resulting in easier erections. "Daily vigorous exercise of moderate intensity and of duration not exceeding 250 minutes per week improves sexual responsiveness and activity."

Drugs, legal and illegal, can cause impotence: cocaine, marijuana, Valium, barbiturates, Tagamet . . . Dr. Flatto gives a five-page list of offending medications, ranging from antidepressants to gastrointestinal drugs and nasal sprays. According to the *Journal of the American Medical Association,* a quarter of male sexual problems are caused or complicated by medication. Once again, good diet and plenty of exercise may be sufficient to restore potency. It is widely acknowledged by the medical profession that many of the drugs we take would be unnecessary if we ate more fruits and vegetables, less junk, and went on a brisk march across the fields a couple of times a week.

Of the more serious physical causes of impotence, prostate disease is the most common. The majority of men suffer from it at some period in their lives, and all men over thirty-five should get themselves examined regularly. The prostate is a small gland at the bottom of the bladder, about the size of a chestnut, whose job is to secrete some of the fluid that makes up semen. It can go wrong in a variety of ways, from mild inflammation to cancer, so it is worth looking after. Yet again, diet and exercise are the key. The actual causes of prostate disease are not yet fully understood, but it seems that zinc deficiency is an important factor. All men of all ages should be sure to eat a good quantity of nuts and seeds, whole grains, carrots, and other foods such as fresh peas (canned peas are not the same thing at all—they have been nutritionally massacred) that are high in zinc. Prostate cancer has also been linked to high-fat diets.

The psychological causes of impotence are problematic because they are vague. However, sex therapy succeeds in about 75 percent of cases. The cause may be psychological if (1) impotence arrives suddenly after a major crisis, (2) it is present with only some partners but not others, (3) the man can still masturbate to orgasm, but can't have an erection when a woman is present. A bad day at work, a nasty letter from the bank, a cruel word from your lover: all can cause a temporary inability, which then feeds on itself. The next time the man attempts to make love, he worries so much about not getting an erection that he ruins his chances. If he'd simply realized that his impotence was a passing phase that most men have to put up with now and again, and that simply doesn't matter, he'd have been perfectly okay. If this sort of impotence ever affects you, show this book to your partner. It is extremely important that women do not make an issue out of impotence. There are many ways of enjoying sex without penetration. The woman is justified in expressing annoyance only if the man suffers more than a week or so, but refuses to seek help.

When impotence is psychological in origin, the first thing you should do is talk about it openly with your partner. All images of tough-guy reticence and priapic ability must be thrown out of the window and replaced by an honest discussion about your worries. Such openness is particularly important because the woman will want to be reassured that you're not tired of her and having an affair with the blond bimbo across the street. Once this point has been cleared up, you'll find that women are often surprised how much a passing bout of impotence can mean to a man. Women don't believe that the essence of masculinity is an iron-hard erection and are perfectly happy for sex to take place sometimes without penetration.

The next thing is to make sure that, whenever sex does occur, you feel comfortable and not under pressure to perform. Start thinking you must get an erection, and you will compound the problem. Concentrate on giving her a really good time, orally or manually, and agree that no demands are made upon your penis (many women will be delighted!). If you do get an erection, don't suddenly whip yourself on top and try to plunge in—the result will probably be that you just lose it again, feel foolish, and have to go back to where you were. Let it be. Let your partner fiddle with you wherever it feels nice, if you want, but stay off the intercourse until you find that an erection is fairly easy again. Even then, approach it in stages.

After a few sessions of satisfying your partner, when you find that your erection happens more readily, allow her to give you manual stimulation while you work on her. Don't expect it to lead to orgasm. Indeed, at first forbid such a thing, so that you don't feel under pressure to perform. Next allow her to orally stimulate your penis. Move on to intercourse—probably several evenings later—only when you feel as relaxed as possible about it. Don't say: "Right, today we're going to do the real thing at last." Just allow it to happen it you feel it's right, and be quite prepared not to do it at all if you still feel hesitant. It is by this gradual, relaxed approach that you will overcome the problem. It may take only a few days. It may be cleared up in one evening. Or it may take considerably longer. But it will work. In the meantime, you will have become a positive star at performing oral and manual sex on women.

There are a variety of good books on the market that discuss this therapeutic approach in more detail. For men who cannot face anything with "impotence" in the title, I recommend Bernard Zilbergeld's *Men and Sex*. It has three chapters on the subject, complete with carefully designed exercises for men with a cooperative partner. It also has a plan for men without a regular lover or with a miserable, unsympathetic fiend. *Making Love,* by Michael Castleman, is much less detailed, but good on consolation and background information. (Mr. Castleman endearingly writes: "My own penis is like everyone else's—a little too small. Not that I think size matters, you understand; but still, an extra inch couldn't hurt . . .") Flatto's *Super Potency* is interesting on diets, and shows how to keep your prostate healthy by a series of stretching and twisting exercises, but, despite its title, it does not contain a useful behavioral program for restoring potency.

There are a host of purchasable remedies for impotence, ranging from the silly to the destructive, including a few that are actually useful. Pills and potions bought in sex shops should be treated for what they are—a joke. No aphrodisiac has ever been found to increase sexual performance, although some of them can have an indirect effect by inducing a fit of giggles, or creating an erotically charged atmosphere. The irrepressible Barbara Cartland exclaims that "Honey is the answer!" If "genital function" is really bad, nonperforming scoundrels are encouraged to eat a special concoction of multivitamins, GEV-E-TABS, mysterious stuffs called Celaton CH$_3$ Tri-Plus (the reason why "last year I wrote twenty-four books"), Keitafo Banlon ("communicated secretly from the Chinese Imperial Palace"), and ginseng—two, one, four, and two tablets, respectively.

Bands strapped around your penis help maintain an erection by forcing the blood to remain in the poor thing instead of flowing in and out as it does naturally. They work badly and will end up damaging the delicate penile tissue, so you'll be worse off than ever. If used too long, gangrene will set in.

Testosterone injections used to be very popular, but are effective only when impotence is due to having low levels of the hormone. Injections of various other substances—including, evocatively enough, nitroglycerine—are sometimes used, but all such measures should be approached with great caution.

Finally, there're implants. These are the last resort, and should be considered only for cases in which impotence is due to an irresolvable physical problem, such as diabetes, prostate surgery, vascular disease, or spinal injury. They are inserted into each of the two spongy chambers that make up the core of the penis and come in a variety of curious types.

The most important thing to remember is that impotence does not mean the end of your sex life. In his book *Any Man Can,* Dr. William Hartman quotes a diabetic called Tim, in his seventies, who became impotent as a young man; yet he regularly had multiple orgasms during oral and manual sex. He even went into Hartman's lab to prove it. "It's foolish for people to think a man has to have an erection for a couple to have good sex." Tim's wife agreed. "We feel our sex life is great. We get together two or three times a week—and it's always as good as this."

8

Fantasy

*W*omen fantasize more than men, and their fantasies are extremely explicit. "A vampire dressed from head to foot in black with an enormous penis, lustfully parting my white thighs." "Animals really turn me on. No games played there. No emotional baggage—just sex because it feels good." "I'm a sought-after love goddess." "Pretending to be a lonely house-wife and having the TV repairman visit you." "It's my first time and it hurts and I bleed. Weird I know." "Submissive, over-powering, little girl (bad), violation, doctors, police, wartime prison camps, bondage, *domination*."

I'm tied down in the dentist's chair with the dentist's wife and assistant (also female) playing with my nipples, clitoris and vagina. I'm going bonkers, but can't quite reach orgasm until the dentist appears, sits between my legs at the end of the chair and makes it tilt *way* back, so my genitals are practically right in his face. He doesn't even touch me, but the thought of him just looking makes me have a long hard orgasm. Things proceed and the three of them do all sorts of naughty wonderful things to me. I don't quite understand this fantasy because I do hate going to the dentist. P.S. It's not even my real dentist in the fantasy—he's a real dork! Did I shock you? Ha! Hope this gets to you and isn't read by some perverted publisher.

Being "taken" against my will, which is something which repulses me in real life but I find the thought of it incredibly stimulating.

When I fantasize it's violent sometimes. Being submissive, overtaken, hit, restrained, all very violently. It worries me.

A big macho guy pounding into me. I like it when he makes animal noises and groans, especially when he comes.

They're really terrible, my fantasies, and I've tried often to do without, but finally gave up and accepted it as a really weird thing about myself.

"I could write a book on all the fantasies I have," exclaims "Reader" from Cincinnati, who has, thankfully, refrained. "Fantasies are a MUST!! They spring from nowhere and only come to mind during intercourse or masturbation—not before or after. Fantasies with more than one partner—with a servant or paper boy—with a priest or a girlfriend's father—people I hardly know that I see on the street, etc., etc.! (I'm embarrassed!) The author Nancy Friday has not refrained. For those of you interested in the subject, her set of fat books in which women's (and men's) sexual fantasies are catalogued in all their variety rest broken-backed on bookstore shelves throughout the country, pored/pawed over by young men who haven't the nerve or the dough to buy the things.

Elaborate fantasies are an obvious enhancement to women's desire for "whole context" sex. We create a situation, a scenario, an elaborate story—a wonderful world of tastes, sounds, smells, sights, textures—and place ourselves in the middle of it. We do it for erotic effect: fantasy is a marvelous way to make the simple act of making love more cinematic. Fantasy expands sex and intensifies it. It makes up for the fact that women have a libido that is as high or higher than men's and yet we find satisfaction harder to come by during sex. Vicky from New Zealand:

> In the last year I've been playing some of them out—like tying my partner up and teasing him, being tied up, being spanked and spanking my partner. Being "forced" to suck my partner's cock while my hands are tied behind my back. There have been periods where I haven't needed a fantasy to have an orgasm but most of the time I'm scared I won't come unless I fantasize.

Reality and fantasy are further apart for women than for men because women are more vulnerable. We have more to lose if sex goes wrong: we cannot stride into interesting sexual situations and make them happen without great risk. It's not, for example, easy to set up a real harem scene where the men are sexually desirable, where you are ravished just the right amount but not too much, and where, when you've had enough, all the men politely pack up and go home. In fantasy we can award ourselves full control of the situation.

Roxanne, a forty-seven-year-old psychiatrist, explains also that "women probably fantasize more and harder than men, because the traditional idea of feminine behavior is a burden to a woman during sex. When you're feeling hot and raunchy and disreputable the last thing you need to be distracted by are thoughts about whether you look feminine, sound ladylike, and all the baggage that women have not yet shed. Fantasy restores the balance. Add to that that women spend more time thinking up stories anyway, and read more fiction than men, and you've got a wild world in there . . . lewd extravagances that I'll bet most men never even come close to imagining!" By focusing on some aspect of sex that she finds particularly arousing, and by exaggerating it to the point of outrageousness, a woman increases her chances of climaxing. It's like a sexual essence distilled by alchemists and sprinkled over the double bed. "I like erotic talk," explains Ann, "as it excites me and has the added bonus of keeping my mind on the job, so to speak." Also there's none of the distasteful side of humankind to put us off: no sweat, spots, garlic fumes, no mutual embarrassment over unshapely tummies when you both strip off and make love in the middle of Carnegie Hall with everybody watching, no saying the wrong things, no premature ejaculation. And sometimes fantasy improves a man we'd really rather not be in bed with: "With this partner fantasies are a big help," writes Michelle. "What sort of fantasies? Well, it doesn't hurt to TRY [underlined three times] to pretend he's Fabio."

Some women are choosy about where they draw their inspiration. One lady began her sex life early when she masturbated to fantasies of Rupert bear. Brenda, a young Southern Baptist, discovered her father's *Playboy* and *Penthouse* collection, while Celia was turned on when she came upon a collection of porn videos under her teenage son's bed. Writes another:

> I like to read erotica . . . Anything: letters to *Penthouse,* erotica by women, true stories, lies. I love to read about varied sexual experience . . . I prefer writing by "smart" people. "I was a crack whore" is NOT my ideal story title . . . My own experience isn't varied enough to work out a realistic scenario. I get stuck on details.

Do a Woman's Fantasies Tell You What She Really Wants?

Sometimes.

When?

When she says, "I dream that I'm making love to a wonderful man on the lawn of a mansion on the Vineyard, totally naked," then you can be fairly sure that if you buy her the mansion, she'll probably oblige by acting out the fantasy. (I'm game myself for that one.) Sex in the kitchen, up a tree, on the 23 bus, behind the sociology shelves at the local library—are all Reasonable Fantasies.

> This is where my dream lover comes in. I can pretend we're on a desert island, in a field full of flowers, even once in a shop window, anywhere at all and it makes it so exciting. I recently went for a flight in a hot air balloon and I thought how wonderful to have made love in the basket while drifting along, what a wonderful thought! I would have done it too given the chance. I'm getting excited just thinking about it now!

This same *How to Have an Orgasm* reader gives a good example of how fantasy can help a marriage that is not ideal. Her dream lover does all that she yearns for her husband to do, and does it very well from her account!

Next comes the Acutely Embarrassing fantasy. The one in which she dreams of being taken unawares in church behind a pew while the hymns are being sung. You *could* act this one out—but proceed with caution. Or at least reserve it for lovers you don't mind not seeing again.

Last comes the Extravagant Fantasy, the most popular of all with women. For Debbie in Australia it's:

> Being a buxom serving wench in medieval garb. Being part of a harem. At the slave markets having sex with a prospective buyer in front of the whole marketplace and everyone getting off on it. A strong, forceful, domineering sexual contender. Suggesting sex to strangers and fucking in dark alleys. Public place sexual encounters.

Here, the only rule to obey is that the more extravagant or humiliating the fantasy, the less she's going to want to carry it out in fact. *Always* assume that violence or force is *out*. Get the wrong idea when she starts describing the more extreme versions of these and you're likely to find yourself in the high-security wing of Alcatraz. That does not mean you cannot play-act: "I've always had wild fantasies about being lashed to the mast of a ship and being taken by a ten-foot Viking" could be translated into "Can you please tie me to the bed (not too tightly), and dress up in a helmet, red beard, and loincloth," although it sounds a poor substitute for Osblood the Terrible.

"I always fantasize about things that would scare the hell out of me in reality," reveals Cheryl, who is writing sitting up in bed.

Being owned, being someone else's sex slave or a family's sex slave (to parents and older children). Being used by, say, the milkman or plumber, etc. Used to entertain guests and family at a party. Used to get a better job by screwing the boss at the place where my "master" works. Being in bed with my master and his wife; having the wife's friends touch me. Being given to the local pastor on Saturdays when the family is out shopping. The different scenarios are endless and some complicated. Another fantasy is being taken by a load of monks at the altar of a church.

Karen, a quiet, shy, self-effacing forty-two-year-old shop assistant, surprised the hell out of me when she told me what her sexual daydream was:

Thank you for asking! Now I can write it down for a reason, on the grounds that I'm furthering human sexual understanding! Setting: a bar. I've run out of money for a drink, so I go up to one of the men sitting by the counter and put my hand on his crotch and ask for the money to get a drink. I don't open his fly, I just rub his pants until he creams and I never take my eyes off him. I know when he's done it because his pants get moist. But then it turns out he doesn't have any money, so I'm angry. I get contemptuous and make fun of him, so all his friends begin laughing at him. He keeps asking me to stop, and I get at him more and tell him the only way he'll get me to stop is if he satisfies me in front of his friends. But his dick's gone limp and so he can't do it that way, so I make him give me oral sex, right there in the bar with his friends laughing and getting all hot. He pulls down my panties and gets under my skirt, then I come and feel the liquid go over his face and I won't let him go until I'm finished completely. But I'm still not satisfied, so one by one I have all his friends too. They have to satisfy me first, but instead of letting them ejaculate in me I make them do it in a glass instead. After I've finished with them I go back to the original one who's hard again by now. I pour Worcestershire sauce in the glass and as he fucks me I drink it down slowly. I call it an Anemic Mary!

I have this idea in my head sometimes two or three times a day, and have to go to the ladies' room and relieve myself.

Safe to say she too would not appreciate a bunch of fellows down at the bar trying to turn her dreams into reality. Like Cheryl, above, most women made a special point of stressing that what they *imagined* was the last thing they'd actually want to *do*. This applies *always and without exception* to one of the most common fantasies women indulge in . . .

Fantasies of Being Raped

> I need fantasy in order to orgasm. Usually I'm being taken advantage of by men who are enjoying my body. I usually just have to let them do what they want with me (mostly involving intercourse, giving them blow jobs)—all sorts of men (taxi drivers, policemen, soldiers, businessmen).

Why do so many of us have them? Scenarios in which the "weak" woman is being sexually dominated are the "single greatest theme," writes Nancy Friday in *Men in Love*. "They enjoy the idea of being 'forced' by male strength to do this deliciously awful thing, made to perform that marvelously forbidden act..." Yet no woman on earth wants to be raped. Obviously not, since "rape" *means* sexual intercourse against your will. Few women wish to be prostitutes, yet being paid for sex is also a vastly popular fantasy. The usual guess in sociological literature is that forced sex allows women to enjoy lust without guilt. I find this an inadequate explanation. If it were true, liberated women would have fewer such fantasies, and women who feel guilty about sex would have more. There is no evidence for either.

My belief is that rape and prostitution fantasies take the anxiety out of attracting men. Instead of worrying, "Am I beautiful, sexy, feminine, alluring enough?" and all that jazz, we *know* he desires us because he is either forcing sex or paying for it. Bingo! In one fell swoop all the typical female tensions go out the window. My idea was reinforced by a delightfully frank twenty-four-year-old Swede who wrote: "I enjoy manual sex if the man does it for himself, if I know he likes it, or if somebody pays me for it. I cannot get an orgasm if I am not sure they like what they are doing. But they wouldn't pay if they didn't like doing it!"

Rape fantasies are the *opposite* of real rape. In true rape the man controls the woman 100 percent. In fantasy rape, the woman controls *everything*. Not only who he is and what he looks like, but what he does to her, each detail of the setting, and of her own responses. Her "rapist" does things *her* way. "Who am I raped by in my fantasies? A very handsome young shiek usually. Occasionally a lean, trim burglar—I guess I'd find that he's James Bond if I put the light on." Sociological experiments have *proved* what all women know, that real and imagined rape are very different things. In one example the researchers got together a sample of women and played them two recordings. The first was of a typical female rape fantasy "in which the woman is in control because she enticed and permitted the man to 'rape' her for her own erotic purposes." The women enjoyed listening to this one. The second recording was of a realistic rape scene. The women loathed it, reacting with intense "disgust, fear, anger, pain, shame, and depression."

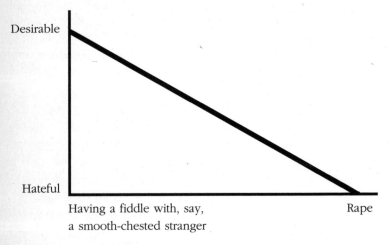

The Interactive Reality-Fantasy Coefficient As Plotted for the Human Female: or, Rachel Swift makes an educated guess about women's dirty thoughts.

Fantasy is a perfect way to see your desires satisfied without the stronger male actually getting out of hand. When the lusty Harlequin hero pinions Arabella to the floor of his racing stables with his passionate rock-hard member, the force is magically delicious. Buggery by King Kong, flagellation with a cat-o'-nine-tails, being assaulted while having your limb amputated on the Napoleonic battlefields (unusual, but often imagined by a demure bank clerk from Trieste, Italy), all lack the cutting edge of real life that would make the actual experience hideous.

At the other end of the scale from rape are fantasies about . . .

Women Dominating Men

The second most common subject for female fantasy, I call these Delilah Dreams (after Samson's friend, the haircutter). Here the woman subdues the stronger male and forces him into all sorts of humiliating situations. The following example arrived on my doormat one fine morning in a purple envelope. It's from Anonymous, "big hips, big tits, big appetite," aged thirty-one, mailed from Lincoln:

> I'm driving alone in the car, desperate for a fuck. I pass the gym where all the men I like are working out. I stop the car across the road and put a dildo, some rounds of rope, rolls of bandages and Vaseline in a duffel bag then go across to the gym. I'm wearing high heels and a bustier. I've got crotchless panties on. The men on the machines—there are three of them—are gawking at me but pretending not to. I make my way around the machines and one by one catch the men out and tie them to the equipment using the rope, before they can get away: one is exposed with his arms raised behind him on the pec machine. Another's clutching the length of the leg exercise bench. The third is lying on his back,

strapped beneath the weights you have to push up above your head. Then I fuck them all. I get on top of number three and push the dildo slowly up his ass while making him say how much he enjoys it. Number two I suck, then make him suck me. I'm quite rough with him. Number one's the man I like most. I sit in his lap, facing him, and force him to lick my breasts. I kiss him passionately when we both climax together. When I'm finished, I leave them tied up. On my way out I pass a group of prim-looking girls going up to the gym to do their exercises.

The sexiness lies in using a woman's greatest strength against a man—her sexual power. The most powerful muscle-bound stranger is reduced to helplessness in three minutes once she draws his penis in between her legs or lips. Such fantasies tend to involve someone other than the real lover: the boss at work, the cruel school principal, the sexy sulky grocer down the road, the ugly toad who lives next door, the boyfriend's best friend . . .

"Oh God!" did I hear you say? Oh God, what? Oh, *that*! You mean . . .

Does She Really Want to Make Love to Your Best Friend?

It depends. How good-looking is he?

Joke.

No. She doesn't necessarily desire the best friend. A recent study concluded that for *unmarried* women the most common fantasy of all during intercourse, masturbation, or just an idle time of day is sex with the boyfriend. Sex with a male friend comes at number seven on the list, and only one in ten of the women interviewed had the fantasy while in bed with their regular partner. Married women, however, are more likely to fantasize about a man other than their partner. One lady wrote to say that she had frequent and very realistic fantasies about other men and "sometimes they were so real it was unbelievable. I used to also encounter the man I had the dream about the very next day, whether I knew him or not, and many times it seemed like they knew about the dream . . ." This curious phenomenon, in which a dream transforms a man from dull dog to sexual magnet, says a lot about the fluctuating nature of female sexual passion. It's happened to me with the actor Oliver Reed, Bill Gates, and (oh shame) an elderly doctor: in each case, at 11 P.M. when I went to bed, the man was highly unattractive, only to be magically transformed into a wild sex symbol the next morning. Luckily it doesn't last. Therefore take warning. If any man notices a sudden change of interest from a woman who yesterday ignored you, there's probably an erotic dream to blame. But work fast if you wish to consolidate the situation. Tomorrow she'll be back to her original opinion!

If your best friend is not the object of a woman's desire, it may well be your sister or her best friend. Fantasies involving sex with other women are extraordinarily popular, even though most of the dreamers insist "I am *straight*." Again and again fantasies involve things that are different from what we want in real life.

> Often they concern meeting up with someone I was in love with years ago, and knowing that he wants me desperately. Or going to a blue film and getting turned on watching another couple nearby masturbate each other. Going pantyless to some public place—I imagine his reaction when he finds out, or I let him know. Letting a lover pee on my private parts (I'm terribly ashamed of this one, would hate it in real life, but it does turn me on).

I often imagined my husband to be a macho man (although I couldn't live with this sort of man!).

Fantasies are very important to me during sex. I'm always thinking them (if not acting them out). They are usually about people I shouldn't be having sex with (a visit to the doctor's/my teacher/my brother—though I don't actually have one). But I also fantasize about other women.

Fantasies of sex with someone whom we know, rather than an attractive stranger, are popular because for women the personal element is important to satisfaction. Doctors are always hot candidates, as are priests, teachers, psychiatrists, and such forbidden figures. Laura, who imagines being ravished by her gynecologist on the operating table, explains her pleasure as "purely sexual. No emotions. I couldn't possibly go for him. He's too old and unpleasant to look at. I would never want to actually kiss him. But somehow the idea's sexy. Because he's the master, in control, or because he's forbidden and I know I never shall?" A strong indication of how divorced this sort of fantasy can be from real life is the number of women who fantasize about their partner making love to someone else. Believe me, if we caught him doing it in real life without our express permission, there'd be murder!

Thinking about someone other than the partner is so common among both men and women that I cannot see it as disloyalty, although some women do: "Fantasies seem like the thin edge of the infidelity wedge" . . . "They make me feel guilty, as if I'm cheating" . . . "When I am with a man I try to make him my focus" . . . "Reality is better" . . . However, at least one woman at the very moment of writing realized that perhaps she'd been mistaken:

Fantasies are all-important during masturbation but I realize that I never go off into fantasy when lovemaking with a partner. Perhaps I'm too busy concentrating on getting it right for him, including tying in with his fantasies, some of which don't exactly appeal to me, and on putting on my own little act. I think I've just found the root of my problem, haven't I? Now how do I change the habits of a lifetime?

Approximately 30 percent of women don't have sexual fantasies. For some, it's a vestige of the old notion that fantasy is something only men do. Others are embarrassed by the harshness of their sexual inspiration and quickly squash it.

Acting Out Fantasies Together

Chris used to love spanking me, and I was turned on by his pleasure, rather than the act itself. John, however, cannot bear the thought of inflicting physical pain on someone he loves, so when he tried to spank me I knew he wasn't enjoying it, so it did nothing for me. I had to explain that it was the thought of being able to fulfill a fantasy that aroused me, not the physical pain.

I like to talk about fantasies before sex. My favorite fantasy is to have another women involved in our lovemaking, or even on my own, but preferably with my partner watching. I love to act out a lover's fantasy: it does not make me feel submissive, rather in control, because they are relying on me for their excitement.

A lot of the time sex is boring. I've always fantasized about two girls and a guy. I have done it before with other people before my husband and lately have thought about it hard. Maybe it will put some spice back in our love life. But you just can't go up to your best friend and say, "Wanna have a three-way with me and my husband?" You could probably lose a friend. Got any suggestions how to bring it up with someone?

If you're acting out fantasies, proceed with care—not everybody likes hearing their beloved's secret lusts. Graham, an eloquent botanist living in Madras, paid no heed to this word of caution on his first night with his fiancée, Annie. "Earlier in the day we'd been talking about what women find sexy and I'd gotten the idea that she liked humiliation. She kept saying how women have fantasies about submissiveness and exploitation, and how this was a real insight into the female psyche . . ."

So I had her down in the role of an impoverished, fearful creature who the big man was going to penetrate in every orifice while she pleaded for mercy and cried bitterly, before discarding her back on the streets. So there I was, describing what I was doing, acting it out and getting a bit carried away, bedsheets flying, so to speak, when Annie suddenly pipes up:

"No, no, not that. Not tears. She's happy about it really!"

Okay, I think, she's happy about it. So I quickly change tack, and say that the tears were all a front, and in fact they are tears of enjoyment. She's so happy about being thrown around, that she laughs joyfully every time he penetrates her with his thick member and every time she laughs her body trembles with the exertion, and her big thighs wobble against his balls squeezing his penis . . .

"Wobble against his balls!" shouts Annie.

"Yes, she's a tall woman," I say, thinking that this will counteract the bad effects of my earlier mistake even more.

"You think I'm fat!"

"No, I think you're gorgeous."

"You want a fat woman—you're in bed with me—you think I'm fat."

"No, honestly . . ."

"I can't believe it. Do you know what size I am? I'm a 12. Right, that's it. Sex is over. Time to go to sleep because tomorrow I get up and start jogging!"

One forty-two-year-old black American thought fantasy was best kept for masturbation. "I don't like fantasies when I'm with a man," she wrote. "I can't see the point. Being with a lover is my fantasy when I'm alone so that when I'm finally with someone it's enough." However, after three years with one lover he began talking about fantasies, and wanted to know what her greatest one was. She refused to tell him. He begged and pleaded and insisted, promising not to get mad, no matter what it was. "I told him (after much urging on his part) that my fantasy was to have sex with a white man . . . He was light-skinned so I thought we could pretend by putting a blond wig on him or something, but he was so pissed off that he stormed out and wouldn't speak to me for days."

Absolute Sizzlers

Absolute sizzlers are, ironically, often sexual fantasies where no sex takes place at all. Women's imaginations are such that often the very context is enough: "I invent a long, slow story beginning with a chance meeting and (theoretically) ending up in torrid sex. But I never *reach* the end. The anticipation is enough to drive me wild."

I can't tell you how sexy inexplicit sex can be. Tantalizing. Sex is like coffee. The smell and anticipation of it is always better than the real thing.

One of the most enduringly popular Absolute Sizzlers is Jane Austen's *Pride and Prejudice,* first published in 1813. The story of a man and woman who meet, wrongly evaluate and therefore despise each other, and maintain an electric sexually charged dislike over three hundred pages, it is certainly the sexiest book I've ever read, though the hero and heroine never even touch. As I write, twelve million viewers are currently enthralled with A&E's TV adaptation. At my local all-girls get-together, sensible married women tell me that Mr. Darcy is so unutterably sexy that they cannot read about him when their husbands are in the same room. Harlequin, publishers of romantic fiction, have built a whole industry on the formula of mutual dislike and sex kept well within bounds.

Even in modern times, some of the greatest erotic moments have nothing overtly to do with sex—no nudity, no grunts and groans, only a devastating erotic atmosphere: Humphrey Bogart lighting Lauren Bacall's cigarette in *To Have and Have Not,* James Mason sizzling with suppressed anger and passion for Ann Todd in *The Seventh Veil,* or the hero and heroine manacled together, hissing at each other for two days in *The Thirty-Nine Steps.*

The last word on the subject, however, must go to the wise Barbara Cartland, seller of six hundred million books that play on women's romantic fantasies:

Sex is important to everybody, but I think it's been blown up into a thing that you must have and must do, and what we're talking about as sexuality today is lust—it's not love. People are told they must rush into bed and do peculiar things off the chandelier, which is a lot of rubbish. The whole thing has been blown up. I was the best-selling author in America when the romantic era came in. I sold something like two million copies of every book I wrote. There was no competition. Then along came these romantic authors who were told to write like Barbara Cartland with pornography. I know them well, they're very sweet to me. They're middle-class, middle-aged women. Half of them have never been kissed, let alone done those filthy things off the chandelier, but they're told it's what sells. That's just nonsense. I sell more than any of them. None of my books are dirty, none of my books are immoral, I don't have pornography in them, and mine sell.

9

Mysteries of the Female Orgasm

Sometimes I think that women are a totally different species, you know, and that I would understand chimpanzees or mermaids better than I understand my wife sexually.

—MARK, TWENTY-SEVEN

Women's orgasms are the most baffling things. With a man, it's simple: a rub or a twiddle or a bit of in and out and bingo! But women? They're like the theory of relativity by comparison. Their vital parts are almost invisible. They can take two minutes or two hours or never come at all. Some say they're satisfied without orgasm, and others want to tear you limb from limb. They claim they can do it twenty times in a row and they've got umpteen different *types* of the thing. It's no wonder that men find women utterly mysterious. Women find themselves mysterious. "I know if I live to be a hundred years old," complained one man, "I shall never, never, never understand what happens to my girlfriend down there. And what is really crazy, she agrees with me!"

Okay, let's begin to demystify the matter.

What Are the Different Types of Orgasm?

Proposing types of female orgasm is something of a sport with sex researchers. From a lover's point of view the best thing is not to worry about it. An orgasm is an orgasm, and very pleasant whatever qualifying label gets attached to it. Nevertheless, the subject excites an enormous amount of attention, and the well-informed man has a certain rarity value.

The two main proposals are the **vaginal** and **clitoral** orgasms. The distinction was "discovered" by Freud at the turn of the nineteenth century, who insisted that mature women have orgasms due to stimulation of the vagina alone, by the penis, whereas immature women can have orgasms only if they stimulate the clitoris as well. He based this distinction on the fact that girls who masturbate almost always concentrate on the clitoral region, without using any vaginal penetration at all, whereas married women climax when they have a man's penis inside them. The idea has since been soundly trashed. Even during intercourse, almost all orgasms are due to clitoral stimulation, because the position of the man's pubic region provides considerable friction to the area. The reason Freud didn't know this is probably because he was impotent for most of his life. When a man enters from behind, thus avoiding such contact with the clitoris, women hardly ever climax except if the act of moving in and out pulls at the vaginal lips and thus excites the region indirectly. Helen Kaplan writes in *The New Sex Therapy,* "regardless of how friction is applied to the clitoris, i.e., by the tongue, by the woman's finger or her partner's, by a vibrator, or by coitus, female orgasm is probably almost always evoked by *clitoral* stimulation. However, it is always expressed by *circumvaginal* muscle discharge."

The discovery of the **G-spot** in the 1950s introduced a new argument for vaginal orgasms, for a few women. First proposed by Ernst Grafenberg, the G-spot is an erotic zone found about two inches inside the vagina on the front wall. Insert two fingers, facing forward, about halfway in and wiggle. At first stimulation of it causes a desire to pee, but this is quickly replaced by sexual arousal and enlargement of the spot, which can lead to orgasm (or multiple orgasms), plus the ejaculation of a large quantity of clear, transparent fluid, similar to semen. For a long time it was suggested that the fluid was urine, but this has now been conclusively disproved. The trouble with the G-spot is that most women don't seem to have one, at least not one that's sensitive. And it's also far from proven that stimulating it leads to a fundamentally different type of orgasm. It is possible, for example, that fiddling with the G-spot is a way of stimulating the clitoral roots, so that the orgasm is still via the clitoris.

The great race to find location-based orgasms could quickly get out of control if people followed it to its logical conclusion. What, after all, is to be made of all the women who climax merely by having their breasts fondled? Do they have bosom orgasms? And do other women have eyebrow orgasms and neck orgasms and teeth orgasms? Some women describe what they call **emotional** orgasms, "an intense emotional feeling flooding all over me. It comes in great waves, has nothing to do with my genitals, and leaves me feeling disturbed yet wonderful." Then there's the matter of **nocturnal** orgasms ("Nocturnal orgasms? Are you kidding?" wrote Lynette), provoked by nothing except erotic dreams. They're delicious, soothing, wild, and . . . "Kind of scary, actually," according to Margie. "You wake up and look over and your partner's sound asleep!" The best thing about them is they happen effortlessly: "No thinking involved, just feeling. Great!" Yet they may involve complications: "Once I dreamed a guy from work was performing anal sex on me," writes M. H. "I was groaning and writhing so much my husband woke me up. Thank God he didn't ask any questions!"

Obviously, women's ability to climax is derived from a center of pleasure in the brain to which there are many roads of access, the main highway being the clitoral system, shaft, and root. Apart from that . . . no need to worry your pretty head over it.

What Is the Point of Female Orgasm?

The point, says the anthropologist/author Desmond Morris, is the survival of the next generation. If a woman has an orgasm during sex, then she is more likely to form a stable "pair-bond" with her fellow, and thus improve the survival chances of the child. But this is only one theory among half a dozen: the reason for female orgasm is an enduring mystery. Some researchers have suggested that the vaginal contractions draw the semen up into the womb and improve fertility; others insist that orgasm has the opposite effect.

The case of the male orgasm is, of course, straightforward, at least in pure survival terms. It is a pleasurable sensation that encourages the man to spill his seed as often as possible. As long as the woman is there to receive the gift, whether willingly or not, the population will increase and there's no need for evolution to bother itself with the matter any further. In short, physical weakness and/or a certain degree of enjoyment on the woman's part are all that's required. Female climax seems to be taking things a little too far. This knotty problem is further complicated by the recent discovery that some female primates have orgasms. In fact, it's believed that many of the higher mammals could enjoy this privilege *if only the males could keep going long enough*. Premature ejaculation is rife in the animal kingdom.

Is It Really True That Women's Sexual Potential Is Enormous?

Yes.

The real testing ground of sexual potential, in both men and women, is masturbation, not intercourse. Masturbation is one of the few instinctive human behaviors that we can study. It is the purest part of our sex life. One writer has called it "*the sexual base*. Everything we do beyond that is simply how we choose to socialize our sex life." Put in practical terms, this means that during masturbation a person can concentrate solely on satisfying her desire, without distractions from a partner. All concerns about him coming too soon, moving badly, or saying something hideously embarrassing just as the floodgates are about to open, are gone. Sex on one's own is rarely as pleasant as it is with a good man, but it is less complicated. It is a time of pure physical hedonism, when a woman can do exactly as she would be done by.

How do women score on this measure of sexual potential? We're incredible.

Over 80 percent of women today admit to masturbating (the precise statistics vary) and nearly all can reach orgasm easily and quickly, usually within a couple of minutes or less:

It takes two minutes. I lock the door (three roommates!), then lean against the wall and watch myself in the glass of the dressing cabinet door. I drop my skirt, pull my panties halfway down my thighs and use the tip of a vibrator against my clitoris until I'm on the point of coming, when I slide all nine inches of it into my vagina and climax immediately.

Orgasm? Every time—always. It's because I have a vivid imagination and always imagine myself with a man. Sometimes with two men.

I've even timed myself; I can have an orgasm 99 percent of the time in less than thirty seconds.

I climax nearly every time I masturbate. I am a master!

I usually masturbate when I'm feeling horny and can reach orgasm quickly (under five minutes). Lately I've chosen to stretch it out, make it last, try different things. Just bought a vibrator and love it.

If I want one I get one. They are different, though— sometimes it will be quick—a snap, instant relief. Others are slow, involved, tortuous . . .

One orgasm is often followed by a second, then a third and a fourth . . . Of those women who've written to me, I calculated that between two and five orgasms each session was a reasonable average, with many women going into double figures.

The range of sensation is also enormous. For some, masturbation does not result in orgasm at all: the best advice for them is to keep trying and experiment with plenty of different positions and methods—showerheads that direct a stream of water at the clitoris are so popular that several women named theirs! In a few women masturbation leads only to discomfort and itching: "Orgasm, smorgasm," remarked Mary, a twenty-seven-year-old accountant. "Don't have one and don't want one. It sounds a messy distressing business to me. I only bought your book because I thought I ought to know a little bit about it. Much rather go hiking."

At the other end of the scale women's capacity is limited only by exhaustion, boredom, or interruption: "Sometimes, once I start the urge just keeps coming back," writes Anstey. "Sometimes I really want another one, but my muscles will no longer contract (arm muscles included!)." Rosemary explained how her husband had bought her some Burmese Bells to keep her occupied while he was away at a conference in France. This ingenious device consists of two connected metal balls, which are inserted in the vagina. One of the balls is hollow and goes in first. The other contains something heavy, such as a smaller ball, mercury, or lead pellets, which will oscillate pleasantly when the user sways her hips. The day before hubby's return, she became so lusty with anticipation that she inserted them before going off to play soccer at her evening class. By halftime she'd lost count of the number of orgasms she'd had (not to mention bad kicks, fouls, and own goals). By the end of the game she was so exhausted that she couldn't bring herself to have sex with her husband until three days later.

Most of the rest of us, however, lie between these extremes:

I orgasm at least once each time. After that the others come easier and quicker. I can time them accurately. Doing it to music, when the volume is on full. Then I sit in my armchair. I throw my legs over the arms so that I'm exposed to the mirror in front and see my pussy getting red, wet. As I come I buck in the seat. I'm on the floor by number six. The music covers up the noise I can't stop myself making.

Usually two. The first being sharp and intense; the second deep, washing all over me, leaving me quivering and very relaxed. Four—once—Wow!

Some of them are really powerful, particularly if it's taken a long time or if I have delayed the orgasm deliberately. One very intense one or three small ones can put me in a good mood for days.

One orgasm is all I can deal with during any session . . . they tend to be a tad too intense.

I masturbate between one and twenty times a week. The frequency varies with the way I feel. If I feel good about myself I seem to do it more than when I don't feel so good about myself . . . it probably has a lot to do with self-confidence.

Record? Fifteen. This was when I was fucking myself in the garden shed. It was like Lady Chatterley. The gardener came in while I had my back against the wall. (I thought he'd gone home and my husband was out.) My jeans were pulled down and my hand was playing with my pussy and my eyes were closed so I didn't see him. When I opened my eyes he was staring. I was too embarrassed to continue, but he made me go on. He knelt in front of me, and sometimes I rubbed myself against his face. Mostly he just watched. I came fifteen times that afternoon. He left afterwards. We fucked on the table, but he didn't insist on it. That made sixteen.

I never am completely satisfied . . .

How do we manage it? Without the mess that men make, or the embarrassing protrusion, it's very simple: in bathrooms or dark corners, under office desks, a little gentle leg-crossing in the bus home from work. In *How to Have an Orgasm* I suggested that to become a master masturbator women should perfect their technique in public or semipublic. Egad! The interviewers were shocked at that. One publisher had even refused the book because of it. But far from being outlandish, many women do so frequently:

Sometimes if the train is busy I like to do it while people are watching. I use the spine of my book or my handbag and take advantage of the motion of the carriage. Mostly I'm more careful. In the bath with the shower spray. That's why I spent three days investigating the best brand of shower!

Horse-riding of course. And before I had my horse I used to love to sit astride gateposts in the country. I was always taking friends on country walks, then I'd innocently chat sitting astride a stile.

The greatest pleasure and challenge when you masturbate in public is to keep a straight face and steady voice when you climax. I've several times been in the middle of talking to someone on the telephone at work, and once when I was doing it under my desk my boss was actually talking to me across the desk.

I have only had an orgasm while standing on my head (I'm really not kidding) so although I *can* do it in public, the circumstances are rather limited!

It's a real game to me. I keep a sort of I-Spy record of all the places I've pleasured myself: art museum, various coffee shops, on the bus, with my dog lying between my legs.

Although women use dildos for masturbation, they are mostly for stimulating the clitoral area—only at the last minute will the object be inserted. All that porno-mag concentration on long, thick penis substitutes such as cucumbers, bananas, candles, brush handles, whiskey bottles, baseball bats, astronomical telescopes, and express trains is misleading. Penetration during masturbation is a side issue for most of us. If your partner is not too inhibited, suggest she satisfy herself in front of you. What she does and the way she moves her hands will give you important clues about what you should be doing to her.

Although women, when they do masturbate, can knock the spots off men, we are more varied in how often we do it. Unlike men, whose desire is fairly evenly spread across the days and months, women oscillate between periods of calm and periods of great lust. To some extent this is due to her time of the month (see chapter 7, "Penetration"); but there is more to it than that. It's context again. Even in masturbation, the circumstances are important. If the context is arousing, we may have uncontrollable desires to do it every hour on the hour for a week. If the conditions are not quite right, or after a bad sexual experience, women can go for a long time without feeling the urge.

> Sexual feelings are delicate. The last time I experienced sexual desire was one and a half years ago. It was the morning that my lover was due to leave my bed to go off to meet one of his other girlfriends, who was arriving to spend two months' vacation with him. Because I knew I wouldn't be able to sleep with this man again for a while and because I have never been able to resist him (we've had four years of an off-on relationship, having a child together, and wonderful sex), I was longing to make love to him. But he left my bed at 7:30 A.M. without offering a thing, leaving me wet and aching in my loins for a full two hours. I suppose he wanted to be fresh for the new arrival. Since then I haven't felt any desire at all. My body just switched off. I wish I could have that morning back. I would force him to make love to me. Maybe then I would want to masturbate again. As it is—I touch myself and feel nothing—absolutely nothing.

> I have been three months without feeling the need. This was after a bad experience at my dorm when my tutor tried it on with me. I was disgusted by him and it made sex dirty. Recently I've just met up with Kieran, a wonderful man who is so attentive. Because the sex is so mind-bogglingly great, I am constantly thinking about him. I'm always wet. I've had to begin masturbating twice a day in addition to our sex life . . . I'm worn out.

Clearly, women's sexual potential is enormous, but variable and sensitive, and much affected by circumstances.

Yet 70 Percent of Women Have Difficulty Reaching Orgasm with a Man

Despite the enormous sexual ability women display when masturbating, only a third of us achieve even a portion of it during sex with a lover. The same woman who will bring herself to climax in three minutes while chatting happily on the telephone may that same evening have a great deal of difficulty after an hour in bed with the man she adores. And the number of women who can get fifteen orgasms in ten minutes of intercourse is very small indeed. This is an astonishing discrepancy, and it goes right to the heart of women's sexuality.

First, the statistics. The 70 percent figure comes from Shere Hite's first report, published in 1976. I favor Hite because her sample was large, fairly randomly selected, and encouraged detailed answers without having a white-coated sex researcher breathing down the respondent's neck. A survey of 4,000 readers of *Woman* magazine came up with even worse results. *The New England Journal of Medicine,* on the other hand, produced a figure of only 46 percent: much more optimistic, but still distressingly poor. (It also noted that one in ten women suffer from having an orgasm too soon—I've yet to meet one of those! I wonder what they're complaining about.) Very recently, Susan Quilliam's *Women on Sex* found a similar result: 53 percent of her sample climax easily, but only one in four women do it all the time during sex.

Shocking though the statistics are, many women have found it secretly comforting to discover they are not the only ones who experience this enormous discrepancy between masturbation and intercourse. For years I was unable to have an orgasm except by masturbation, and assumed I was a freak. I remember the relief when I discovered Hite: after reading her report a personal difficulty turned into a crusade. What's more, it's getting better for all women. We're more sexually confident than ever before, and men are more considerate lovers than they used to be.

But a word of warning. I know of men who, on hearing these statistics, seize upon them as a means to deny responsibility when their partner doesn't climax. "Oh well," they say, sounding relieved, "it's obviously not my fault." This is lousy logic. Poor lovemaking is still one of the most important causes of orgasm difficulties.

Why Do Women Have Such Difficulty Climaxing with a Lover?

There are three possible answers to the problem.

1. There is something physically wrong with the woman that may make sex painful and unenjoyable. But even though women who don't climax are often convinced that "I've got a vital part missing," etc., physical causes for long-term lack of orgasm are rare.

2. The man is not performing properly: climaxing too soon, stimulating the wrong parts, being rough, making the woman feel under pressure to perform. This is extremely common and often means that the woman doesn't even enjoy herself, much less climax. Chapter 11, "Orgasm: Women's Practical Advice to Men," discusses the subject in detail.

3. Finally, most frustratingly . . . something else. In *How to Have an Orgasm* I called this something else "The Problem of the Invisible Barrier." It is an umbrella term, covering a multitude of subtleties, but the result is always the same: even when the man is doing everything right for two hours solid, and *the woman is* *highly aroused,* she still can't climax. As soon as she's alone, however, she can usually satisfy herself with ease. Lorraine is an ebullient, buxom thirty-two-year-old who works in Europe as a freelance fashion photographer (you've probably seen a couple of her pictures, without knowing it). She describes a holiday fling in Greece:

> I'd just finished an assignment doing male models for a calendar, and they were in my dreams all the time. I was having nocturnal orgasms a lot, as you can imagine. In the day one or the other of them would come (!) back into my mind and I'd have to go off somewhere, or just stand beyond waist height in the sea, and get rid of the ache in my groin. Then I met this New Zealander who put my models to shame, he was so dishy. He wore bathing trunks like cycling pants, very clingy on tight, rounded thighs. I could hardly breathe when I saw him. When I lay across his groin I thought I was going to explode in seconds. Nothing happened. I was screaming with it I wanted him so bad. I was scratching his face and biting his arms, humping him like a piston. I was wild. I couldn't come, I just couldn't do it.

"It's like you're so close but so far away," said another woman. "It's like you've got all the ingredients you need, but the dish won't come together." Anonymous from Kentucky writes: "My partner feels certain that I have orgasms. In fact, he thinks he's giving me multiple orgasms. How can I be so passionate— laughing, moaning, screaming—and not climax?"

What happens between self-stimulation, which gives so much pleasure, and the stimulation a woman gets from an attentive lover? The stimulation may be excellent in both cases. The only thing that changes is that another person comes on the scene. It's the difference between total control and partial control. The more "in control" of what goes on in the bedroom women feel, the better success they have with orgasm. This is one of the reasons why the difficulty often cures itself as women get older and more confident about pleasing themselves.

The only faintly helpful analogy I can give to describe the subtle feeling of loss of control that some women have during sex with a man concerns speaking on the telephone. Imagine an intimate conversation when you are alone in the room: no inhibitions. Now imagine that your mother or your best friend comes in and sits opposite you. You may not actually be saying anything embarrassing or personal to your partner on the line, but nonetheless you feel inhibited by the third person present. You are no longer wholly in control of the situation.

The problem cannot be discussed briefly—that's why I wrote a 250-page self-help plan explaining how a woman can teach herself to get over it—but there are several ways men can help. First, make sure she feels completely at ease whenever you make love, and do not in any way put pressure on her to climax. Second, encourage her to speak up as much as possible about what pleases her. Submissiveness in bed is one of our sex's most annoying characteristics: don't let her get away with it. Have amnesties where you both agree to be frank about what you like or don't like. Occasionally a woman is too selfless, too distressed, too young, or too cautious to plead her cause, so proceed sensitively. The following is NOT the right way to go about it. Cheryl:

> I had a very insensitive first encounter. I was head over heels in love (love sick). He was the first man I ever had. I'd read loads of sexy mags and books. I thought it was really going to be something. It wasn't. I thought and felt a letdown to him. Sex got no better. I was too shy and didn't know enough to ask him to do what I liked and I didn't want to masturbate in front of him be-

cause I thought he'd think it was dirty and immature. After a couple of months he finished with me. He'd gone on leave and slept with an old girlfriend to find out if he could make her come. Since he had, he said it proved that it was my fault. I felt a wreck. Useless, degraded and dirty. I always feel that it's my fault.

Whose Fault Is It When a Woman Doesn't Climax?

If the man's not sufficiently attentive to allow a woman to climax, then it is, by definition, his fault. If he gives less than fifteen minutes of stimulation (oral, manual, or penetration) or is critical or otherwise selfish in bed, then he is entirely to blame if sex is not up to par for her. Note that the ogre in the above quote managed to prove only that he was up to the job for one woman, but not for another.

If the man is trying his best, however, the only time it is the woman's fault is when she persistently fails to indicate what she likes. Even the most selfless lover needs some feedback.

In a healthy relationship, as long as you are both doing your best, the notion of fault is redundant: *abolish it.* "There is no such thing as an uninvolved partner in a marriage where sexual dysfunction exists," assert Masters and Johnson in their famous (and unhappily titled) book *Human Sexual Inadequacy.* In other words, if one of you has a complaint, then both of you have a difficulty. Remember: men's sexuality is very different from women's and that all that is wrong is that the two of you have not yet reached an understanding. "Fault" does not exist. You may as profitably blame the cat for having a long tail, as your girlfriend for failing to climax. Fortunately, the number of understanding men has increased greatly since the dark days of the 1950s, when sex was considered purely a man's business. Nowadays sensitive lovers are well aware of the role they play:

Gabriel has NEVER implied that my lack of orgasms is my fault. He has in fact understood it as being his fault. I've tried to explain that fault is to be found in our upbringing, in society, in our culture and largely in my head. He still thinks it's his fault. I don't feel that not having an orgasm is my fault exactly—it's not something I am (not) doing and it's not the way I look but I do think that my conditioning and perception is to blame. It's difficult to separate "actions" from "conditioning."

A common practice among men is rushing to disclaim responsibility even when no one is seeking to blame them, which is the coward's way. Others do it indirectly:

I have not been blamed directly, but it sure has been hinted and implied.

My lover has never implied that it was my fault, but he has implied that it was not his own fault.

In fact, women are more likely (and unfairly) to blame themselves than blame their lovers. Resolve today that fault and blame go on the compost heap. They do considerable harm indoors.

What Type of Woman Doesn't Climax?

Absolutely any type.

It's the question everybody wants to know the answer to, and studies on the subject are as plentiful as blackberries in autumn. There's no evidence that religious backgrounds create difficulties: just the opposite in one study, which revealed that churchgoing Englishwomen found orgasm easier than the nonchurchgoers! There is not even evidence, curiously enough, that sexually abused women have more difficulty. Lack of orgasm doesn't mean a woman hates men or is a secret lesbian or wants to be subjugated by male force or any other of the multitude of psychobabble explanations, though some of these may play a part: it means just that she can't come with a man inside her. Sometimes it is a problem only with one particular man—and, maddeningly, he may be the love of her life.

Women of every description, with good lovers to attend to them, have confided to me their difficulties with orgasm: young, old, thin, fat, rich, poor, happily married, nastily divorced, giants, midgets, and mermaids. To take an example, there is the woman who has been married for over twenty years to a man who successfully treats men with sexual difficulties. She is well aware of the irony of her situation and says that, "though my marriage tended to be good . . . I had to suppress my frustration." She thoroughly recommends the services that computer sex has to offer women. Then there is Victoria, a young Korean American:

> I am a friendly person with a lot of friends. I'm popular and I just have a good self-image. I'm about twenty to thirty pounds overweight but proud of every extra inch. I'm proud of myself and of who I am, so I'm not depressed about anything. But . . . I have a problem that I haven't told anyone. I can't get an orgasm by having sex with a man. I can get an orgasm easily and many times by using something that vibrates on my clitoris. (When I'm alone, better if I'm watching an adult film.) Using a dildo, or using something that penetrates me doesn't make me get an orgasm when I masturbate. But don't get me wrong, I love when a man's penis enters me and I love sex. But when I'm with a man I just can't get an orgasm for nothing.

Two things are worth mentioning. There is evidence that a woman's childhood relationship with her father may have some influence. Those who had a reliable and interested father may be more likely to climax without trouble than those whose father was absent or who took little interest in them. The suggestion is inadequately researched, however. But after much consideration about the subject of female orgasm, I believe it is a profitable line to pursue.

Second, it seems that the earlier a woman starts to masturbate, the more likely she'll find coital orgasms easy. John Nicholson, author of *Men and Women: How Different Are They?*, writes:

> Many sex researchers have now come round to the view that the pattern of an adult's sex life is set by his or her adolescent experience of masturbation, and that the reason why men are more sexual than women is that boys masturbate more than girls in the years before they start having sexual relationships with other people. Before they reach adolescence there is very little difference between the sexes in sexuality.

This is probably too strong. The main reason men and women differ in their sexuality is because they are different sexes, a fact that starts to have significant erotic effect only at puberty, when all the peculiar hormones begin circulating in the body. However, masturbation is a very significant part of a person's sex life and forms the core of all the effective modern sex therapy programs, so it would not be surprising if the childhood experience of this innocent pastime had some influence over adult responsiveness.

To end the matter, here is a more curious problem at the other end of the scale. Melissa is thirty-nine years old, an avid biker, and "the type of person who says what's on my mind and if people don't like it that's their problem . . . I don't have a problem with orgasms but I still have an unsatisfied feeling no matter how many I have."

Orgasm Difficulties Don't Mean There Is No Place for Men in Women's Sex Lives

Many men respond with genuine dismay to the 70 percent statistic. It comes as a shock to realize the extent of the difficulty and, by implication, how many women must fake their orgasms or at least imply that all went well when it didn't.

Others find women's success at masturbating threatening. One fellow I know noticed that his wife had become obsessed with taking baths at all hours of the day and night. He crept up on her and caught her in the act with "Rudolph"—her showerhead. He was so jealous that he sulked off and wouldn't sleep with her for a month in pique. Grousing to me, he said, "When Jenny masturbates she can make herself come ten or twelve times in the space of half an hour. She's never climaxed with me, not once, and yet we seem to hit it off well enough, and she's never complained. I feel angry and redundant."

Jenny was astounded by his reaction. "Does he think I *want* it to be that way? It's not so nice for me, either. But until we can both relax about it and learn together to make it work, what can I do? He must slow down and pay attention to what I want him to do to me. All this unpleasantness makes it harder. It brings in an air of recrimination. Anyway," she added, "he ought to be thankful for Rudolph. He gives me at least some outlet, and until we both improve our skills, it saves the relationship from a sexual point of view."

Women masturbate because it is pleasant, and often necessary. An awful lot of us would much rather have the same sensation with a man. Twenty years ago our negative feelings about it were largely due to guilt and a feeling that it represented selfish behavior. Nowadays, our bad feelings about masturbation more often stem from the fact that we miss our partner's company. "I enjoy it physically," is a typical response. "It's a quick release till I get the real thing. Psychologically, no. I still want and need to be touched back, to be licked, nibbled on, talked to, feel the penis pounding inside, and to do the same to the other."

> I much prefer to have a partner. The presence of another body and another's attention feeds my psychological need for love and acceptance.

> Orgasm during masturbation is a quick fix, takes the edge off till later. Sex with my partner is more fulfilling and my orgasm is harder and longer.

> Penetration enhances and prolongs the sensation. It is much more fulfilling.

> Having an orgasm with someone else is a *memorable* experience. In contrast, an orgasm due to masturbation is just run-of-the-mill: still very enjoyable but not the same kind of savoring quality.

> Masturbation is enjoyable physically almost always, but sometimes it just makes me feel more lonely and depressed.

Learn to give your lover what she needs and masturbation will no longer be an issue. Neglect her requirements, and she'll have to get release in any way she can.

Do Women Really Need Orgasms during Sex?

Heavens, yes!

In good sex the physical and emotional buildup is enormous. It begs for release. However, men sometimes don't realize this because women don't have a useful on/off sexual arousal object to indicate that they are still unsatisfied. No woman can ever forget that a man needs sexual relief, because he's got a large and prominent erection to nudge her in the ribs and say "Hey! Don't forget about me!" There are very, very few women, especially nowadays, who don't mind not having orgasms during sex, although the range of their concern varies enormously. Women, though it does not obviously show, may be desperate for sexual relief.

> I would have orgasms all day if I could. I already masturbate nearly twice a day, every day, for more than one orgasm usually.

> Orgasms? They're all right. Quite nice. But you know what I like even better? I like the way a man quivers when he spurts. I like feeling him go limp inside me. It gives me a feeling of great power.

> I used to think orgasm was overrated because I enjoyed sex even without it. But now I am sure that there is indeed a great deal I am missing out on. I don't accept anything else in my life as make do—so why should I accept two-thirds of a sex life just because I feel it would be the easiest option?

> When I do mind I get bitchy and cranky . . . I think most men are selfish pigs, including my husband. And life ain't happy 'less momma's happy!!!!

At the very least, it is impossible for women to forget about the subject. In our society, orgasm is a major issue, constantly reinforced by films and books that show women having them at the touch of a magic button. Put more bluntly: "I'm fed up with saying, 'orgasms are not the goal of sex.' If they are for him then why not for me?"

Complaints about lack of orgasm divide into three types. First, sexual frustration, which speaks for itself. Second, the embarrassment, especially with a new lover and especially nowadays when everyone is aware of the subject. If a woman tells the man at the outset that she's never climaxed, she risks the dreaded "*I'll* make you come" swagger. Third, there is the principle of the thing—something I minded about enormously. Here is an exquisite aspect of life that I was mysteriously excluded from. It takes a saint to remain unmoved when your lover, night after night, year in year out, lies in blissful satisfaction beside you.

> I used to dismiss my orgasmless sex as being blown out of proportion. I enjoyed myself so what did it really matter? But I realize now it does matter to me and my partner because it stops us from feeling equal in experience and we both blame ourselves deep down. I don't want it to become a reason for a rift and therefore feel the need to lie to keep the peace as we are honest about everything else.

Orgasm is not vital to every woman every time she has sex: we vary enormously in our needs. But *orgasm is vital to women as an option*. It becomes a distracting issue only when women want it and are deprived of it. Countless relationships have floundered because the man has not paid sufficient attention to this difficulty and the woman has tried to suppress her frustration by misleading him to think everything is okay.

> I don't mind if I don't set out to try, I am not disappointed. If I do try and become aroused but "fail," I weep uncontrollably when I realize I'm not going to climax—very messy and a negative note on which to end what should be loving and enriching sex. I could more easily avoid sex.

A woman whose partner doesn't show sufficient concern for her own satisfaction, paying attention to her needs as she directs, feels tense, cheated, angry, and unhappy.

When you can't climax, orgasm becomes a terribly important issue. It can obsess you, make you feel terrible. Once you know you can do it, it assumes normal proportions again, as one pleasant aspect of your life.

Recently I told my husband that after eleven and a half years of marriage I'm sick of him being satisfied and me being denied satisfaction. I'm rather resentful.

There are times when I prefer not to think about the fact that he has an orgasm every time and I never do. I'm tired of hurting him by telling him once again that I did not have an orgasm. He usually never asks anymore. When it *does* bother me, I simply want to get away from him, go pee, and put my clothes back on—act like it didn't even happen.

I asked my *How to Have an Orgasm* readers if they were embarrassed to buy the book. The answers were occasionally delightful—"Yes, because they'll think I'm a horny old tramp"—but the great majority of women said they were embarrassed because it suggested they were a "failure."

Most of all, lack of orgasm compounds men's greatest complaint against women. It makes us *not want sex*.

My difficulty with orgasm makes me less enthusiastic to have intercourse with my partner. Certainly when I have a "successful" orgasm I do feel more positive towards life and a greater sense of control.

If I were more confident that I would achieve orgasm I would enjoy the company of men more without feeling threatened and I would have more partners and sexual experiences. I feel it does affect my attitude to men—I distance myself. I put up a protective front.

Yes, it makes men seem so selfish, all of them. Which I

realize is not strictly fair, but that's what it does to you. Just the other evening I was being hit on at a party by an attractive guy. But then I thought: what's the point, and gave him the brush-off.

Definitely. I'm not interested. I don't want to satisfy my partner if he can't satisfy me.

A woman must feel that if she wants to climax you will do your best for her:

Sometimes I get a lot of pleasure simply from pleasing my partner, and sometimes if he's been particularly attentive I just feel so loved and contented that I don't need orgasm. When I do mind, I mind very strongly indeed. There are times when I am so desperate for release that I burst into tears when he comes. (He hates that.) I resent the fact that he can go to sleep and I can't. I've had a lot of sleepless nights in my twenty-three years of marriage.

If I feel I want to please him I don't mind not having an orgasm. I enjoy watching him and the control that gives me. At the times that I am really highly aroused and I don't get an orgasm I mind a lot. It leaves me feeling angry and used and I can't sleep.

A man should *assume* that his partner would like to climax during sex. Don't make an issue out of it by promising you'll "make her come," or pounding away for three hours until she's sore. Read chapter 11 and quietly do your best. Learning to have an orgasm was a landmark for me. It did not change my life, but it made me much more tolerant of men and much more interested in sex.

The Tyranny of Love

How can love by tyrannical?

> My second ever lover [writes Judith], the first man I had
> a proper relationship with . . . told me that an orgasm
> was "90 percent love and 10 percent friction," i.e., if I
> didn't have one, I didn't love him. I was very inexperi-
> enced, he was older than me, more experienced, and I
> believed every word he said, more fool me. I was pet-
> rified of losing him, so began to fake. I must have been
> pretty good, as he believed me until I finally realized I
> didn't need him and told him the truth.

Some people still believe that, as long as the relationship is
close and loving, orgasm will naturally follow. This is a nice
idea but wrong. It is perpetuated by moralistic sex manuals that
offer nonsensical advice such as: "Lie back, relax, love your
partner, and orgasm will be yours." The sad result of this is that
love is used as a form of accusation. "No orgasm? Obviously
you don't love me."

The fact that a woman doesn't climax says absolutely nothing about what she feels for her partner. Many women actually
feel more sexually inhibited with somebody they are close to,
precisely because they are worrying so hard that it'll be interpreted as a failure of love not to climax. A woman's distress at
lack of orgasm is often less to do with her sexual frustration and
more to do with her sadness that it hasn't "set the seal" on her
love.

A close loving relationship may be the ideal situation for
sex, but that doesn't mean women can't enjoy orgasms without
love. Nita is a withdrawn, moody twenty-three-year-old with
such beautiful extremities that she works as a hand and foot
model.

Just when I was beginning to get the hang of orgasm I met a man—can you believe it?—who'd had some bad first experience and who took ages to ejaculate. It was just as if he was a woman—needed long slow buildup and concentration. It was exactly what I needed at that time. He was no great shakes otherwise, but I'll never forget him!

It is not at all uncommon for women to climax for the first time with a complete stranger, or in the most *un*lovey-dovey circumstances.

I've only had one orgasm in my life with a man. A long time ago I had sex with this ugly boy, whom I didn't really want to have sex with, and he made me have an orgasm. It was one time and at first I just wanted to get it over with. It shocked the hell out of me 'cause I didn't expect it. I haven't ever seen him again.

The only orgasm during intercourse I had was when a black Catholic priest I was studying philosophy with forced himself on me with *great finesse.*

Why did I find it easier with a stranger? Because I felt utterly free for the first time. He knew nothing about me. What had I to lose? I couldn't disappoint him, he couldn't judge me.

Ottilie, who is Swiss, was married for sixteen years without an orgasm. She took a lover secretly and learned to climax within two weeks. The love affair eventually petered out because she preferred to use her newfound skills with her husband.

When She Really Doesn't Mind about Orgasm

Orgasm is essential as an *option*. Many women need one every time they have sex, but many are content with only sometimes. Orgasm, like love, should not become a tyranny. That's why I say repeatedly to men, do your best and don't make an issue out of it. There is a fine line between helping lovers to achieve orgasm and simply adding to the pressure on women that already exists. "I like it when a man keeps lovemaking light, not too serious," writes Tanya, fifty-one. "It should be something between friends instead of all this goal-orientated stuff like 'Have you come?' 'Why don't you come?' 'I'm a bad lover if I can't make you come,' which is all so annoying. A lover—of either sex—*must* make it clear that my enjoyment is as important as his/hers, but he/she *must not* make it heavy weather. I've got to have a way of saying stop, go on, do this without feeling somebody's ego's going to get hurt."

> I can thoroughly enjoy giving my partner enjoyment and neither need nor want to have an orgasm myself. My experience has been that this is difficult for my partner to believe or understand. But it is certainly true for me. When I do mind, I usually say so and do something about it.

> Sex can be great without orgasm. I'd like to experience it because I hear it's pretty incredible, but if it's some strange act of God that I'll never reach orgasm—I'm not going to let something so incidental in the grand scheme of things of love and lovemaking make me miserable.

> Orgasms are the frosting on the cake of life. Even if I didn't get the frosting (my favorite part of course) the sex can still be good.

Good sex does not always have to end in a climax for every woman, because the great pleasure of sex is much more than this single experience—it is the whole range of sensations during the act. Accept it as one of the differences between men and women.

Simultaneous Orgasms

Simultaneous orgasms are supposed to be a beautiful symbol of mutual devotion, total equality, and the last word in successful sex. For this reason they're a (rather tedious) necessity in literature and film from D. H. Lawrence downward.

In fact, simultaneous orgasms are wildly overrated. Calculating two people's sexual arousal can be seriously distracting for a woman. The occasions are legion when she's about to come, is teetering on the brink . . . and, three seconds too soon, he comes. Then he's lucky if he escapes in one piece. If you are keen on doing it together, keep quiet about it and look after the timing yourself. It is far easier for men to do this than it is for women. Joy:

> Simmys are good when they happen. I enjoy feeling us going over together, like one flesh. But you don't want to have to think about them. It's a pain. You think: "I'm coming, I'm about to come . . . Oh, better not, he doesn't seem there yet. Better hold back." Result: sex is an exam.

Then, on the odd days when you reach bliss together, you feel quite smart about it.

When you climax separately it's best, for obvious reasons, to let her go first. Then, when your time comes, she can have the extra, somewhat malicious, and thoroughly sexy pleasure of watching you go through the same uncontrollable writhing and groaning as she has just done. Simultaneous orgasm diminishes this. You're so distracted by the feelings in your own body that you can't properly relish the behavior of your partner. "They're not for me," remarks Georgina, thirty-three. "I like to see a man squirm."

Another excellent reason to climax separately is that if the man keeps thrusting while his partner comes, it may result in her having multiple orgasms. Certainly it's true that continued penile thrusts after a woman climaxes can be extremely pleasurable.

Multiple Orgasms

Again, don't worry about them. If you can give her one climax, you've fulfilled your dues and proved your worth. Adding the extra numbers is more a display of her skill at having orgasms than an indication of your special powers. And repeated attempts to make us perform like a bonfire night of fireworks soon become annoying.

Actually, "multiple orgasm" is a term used loosely to cover two different types of climax. A true multiple orgasm is the exclusive ability of a few rare, fortunate women (myself not included). It means a rapid, ungovernable succession of climaxes with hardly any break at all between them and is, no doubt, blissfully exhausting and probably a little scary the first time around. It has much more to do with the physiological makeup of the woman than the quality of the sex. Sequential orgasms are calmer. In sequential orgasms, there is a period in between each climax, of anything from a few seconds to an hour, during which the sensations first cool off and then build up to a crescendo again. They're what a lot of women have during masturbation.

For those of you who are intent, however, the trick with multiple orgasms is not to let there be a lull in movement after the woman's first climax. Unlike men, a woman doesn't have a refractory period during which she has to stop intercourse after coming, so continued stimulation while she's in her most aroused state means that other orgasms (if she wants them) will follow as quickly and as easily as possible. If you wait, it will take much longer because she'll have to build up to a climax from scratch again. That's not necessarily a bad thing, of course, except that, because of all the rubbing and grinding, sex that goes on too long can be painful or boring. Often the woman may also want a change in pace or depth of penetration after her first orgasm, so you should pay attention to what she says and the way she moves:

> My first one kind of exhausts that way of getting there. If I needed slow, careful movements up to that time, I'll want hard, quick fucking for the second one. It's not a big issue, though. If my husband is too aroused to do it and comes, I'm not bothered. It's not a numbers game, it's about mutual pleasure, and after one I'm well pleasured, I'll say!

Note that last remark. Not all women pine for multiple orgasms. The great majority of us are completely happy if we get just one.

10

Faking

I may not be a great actress but I've become the greatest at screen orgasms. Ten seconds of heavy breathing,
roll your head from side to side, simulate a slight
asthma attack and die a little.
—CANDICE BERGEN

*E*very night, hundreds of thousands of women fake their orgasm. As many as 50 percent of women have faked an orgasm at some time.

Why do women fake so much? Do they enjoy being de-
ceitful? Are they secretly mocking their lover's virility? Men understandably feel nervous about the issue, but when a woman
fakes, it is rarely an aggressive act. It is almost always a gesture
of generosity or of defense. She is putting on a performance to
make life simpler for both of you. Remember this simple fact:

NO WOMAN WANTS TO HAVE TO FAKE AN ORGASM.

Everything else follows from it.

How Can You Tell If She's Faked?

You can't. That, from our point of view, is the great beauty of
it. Women's visible responses during sex vary so much that
there is no way to prove whether or not an orgasm has been
faked unless you get down on your knees with a flashlight at
the exact moment and attach a battery of measuring instruments
to various critical parts of the vulva. Erect nipples, flushes, vaginal contractions—none of these is a reliable indicator for all
women. I'll give you an indication of the range of types: among
native tribes, the Choroti women spit in their lover's face, the
Trukese customarily poke a finger in the man's ear, and the Ap-
inaye woman may bite off bits of her man's eyebrows and nois-
ily spit them to one side during orgasm. At the wild end for
Western women is the hot screaming porn-movie orgasm. Some
women really do respond like this, as Anita describes:

> When I'm coming I just lose it. I scratch and bite. It's a
> demon in me trying to get out. I'm uncontrollable and
> shout so loud that everyone can hear; it's very horrible
> but I can't stop because I feel ripped to shreds.

> Oh, fuck, you're telling me, my orgasms are the most
> intense sensations I've ever experienced. The other
> night I was with J. and he said I was like a wild animal
> and afterwards I began crying. The exhaustion of it!

Certainly women are more vocal when they climax than
men are. Then there are the orgasms that might not be orgasms
at all:

> We were on the couch—I was sitting on the couch and
> I was straddled on top of him. He was kissing my
> breasts through my clothes. I *really* love that and we
> were knocking our pelvises together. I felt my arousal

build and build and build and build. Suddenly I felt satisfied. No warm feeling. No electricity. No big bang. No circles of pleasure. Just a calm, satisfied feeling. I was no longer aroused. I felt very relaxed. No fireworks leading to relaxation. No ecstasy. Just a gradual feeling of satisfaction following escalating arousal.

At times my orgasms are little "blips."

Lastly there are the comatose orgasms. In *The Carnal Prayer Mat,* Lady Fruit Blossom after five hundred thrusts finally achieves success: "Starting with her hands and feet . . . [she] began to grow cold, her eyes became glassy, her mouth hung wide open, her breathing halted, all movement ceased and she lay still as a corpse." For fifteen minutes! Enough to scare the daylights out of any lover. This is rare, and even women are inclined to doubt it. The husband of Elaine claims his first girlfriend was so enamored of his lovemaking that she had a fainting orgasm. "It doesn't sound so enjoyable to me," remarks Elaine. "Sounds to me like she was faking."

"Men who worry about faking," observes Henrietta, "divide into two types: nipple men and fluid men. Nipple men check your tits. Every half minute they're checking around to see if the red parts are poking out in an acceptable fashion. Then they say: 'You didn't come. You weren't erect. You don't love me anymore. Oh God!' Or else they're down between your legs with a hydrometer. 'You're not wet. You think I'm a terrible lover! Oh God!' I say: 'I am a woman. I don't get erections. I don't ejaculate!' They don't believe me. I *know* they can't tell because all these so-called fake orgasms of mine are real. I've never pretended in my life. They've always been real ones."

For the most part men can't tell the difference between whether you're in pain or pleasure, so who thinks they can really know whether you've orgasmed or not? If you start squirming or moaning they either stop, or ask if you've had one or just keep going.

I have had a couple of men tell me they could tell if I ever faked it or not. So I tried it and not one of them could tell. And I never told them. And as for going to bed the first time and being able to tell, it's bullshit. They only wish they could. All you have to do is work the right muscles and groan a little and act a little excited. And presto, they think you had one hell of an orgasm.

Women are less likely to fake in long-term relationships. There's less pressure on them to come, and less awkwardness if they don't. However, in long-term love affairs, a different kind of "faking" occasionally takes place. Ruth, a trainee hairdresser, once in a while has to "fake" her orgasm even while she's having a real one. "There are days when orgasm doesn't move me that much. I feel climactic, then glow all over, like a seeping away of all the sexual forces. I don't feel outrageous. I have to pretend it, though. Julian thinks women always make a noise. So I moan loudly, scratch his back, say stupid things, so he knows I'm having what I'm having even though I wouldn't express it that way otherwise."

Juliette remarked, "I tend to be quiet when I climax so I like to add a bit of top-dressing to it. Men expect it. They've watched all that porn stuff where women writhe and scream—and so I provide the goods." Heather:

My orgasms vary a lot. Some days I can't help really yelling; I make an awful racket. The next night I might get one just as pleasurable but quiet and deep. Then I worry Sam'll think I didn't come. Or that I'm not enjoying it. So I soup it up a bit. Actually it's quite fun.

Paige had an unusual theory: "I figure maybe if I fake it, I'd accidentally have one (you know, kind of like visualizing having something you really want)." The idea actually worked for Brenda, who wrote, "I have faked but it usually gets me so excited that I stop faking and really orgasm."

How Do Women Fake?

> After years of practice my faked orgasms are perfect
> and they come in a range of styles to suit every mood.
> Passionate for a stranger or a "makeup" fuck; subdued
> for "post–romantic meal" fuck; funny for a one-night
> stand or silent for that emotional partner.
> —KIRSTY

As soon as women realize how easy it is to fake an orgasm convincingly, they also realize that there are an enormous number of ways in which to do it. Essentially, the results divide into two types: the Silents and the Cecil B. DeMilles. The Silents are sins of omission. When Mr. Man asks that old chestnut, "Did you come?" Miss Woman merely nods, gives him a hug, or smiles smugly. Mr. Man believes what he wants to believe. This is the pleasantest way to fake, requires no energetic attempt to deceive, is probably the commonest, and, I'll bet, practiced even by the most virtuously self-declared nonfaker. As Ann shrewdly remarked: "Ah, let's split some hairs. I'd say I never fake, but I have let lovers think I've come when really I've just gotten very excited. The sounds and movements I make under those circumstances aren't dramatically different from the real thing. Sometimes I know I'm not going to come no matter how long he pounds away; letting him think it happened is the easiest way out."

> I frequently breathe heavily and moan—that might be
> construed as faking an orgasm. Sometimes I don't make

any noise at all. Since my husband and I don't really talk about my orgasms anymore, I'm not sure what I am doing with my moans and groans.

I don't know where Alan got his sex education from. It's certainly peculiar. Every time I feel him ejaculate I smile at him. He thinks that means I've come. I haven't come, but there's no harm in letting him believe I have. I like to think of him satisfying himself and all that hot semen in me. Sometimes I come properly afterwards, and he thinks I've had two orgasms. It's sweet.

The Cecil B. DeMilles come (as Kirsty, above, made clear) in a huge range of types to suit all moods and circumstances. They may be improvised on the spur of the moment, thrown in to coincide with the man's orgasm for maximum camouflage, or practiced in privacy at an earlier date: "I learned to fake by masturbating first," wrote Tammy, twenty-one. "I lay down on the bed with a tape recorder. I pleasured myself with my dildo for *half an hour* until I was nearly flipped and the bedcovers were soaked with juice. It gave me a great opportunity to 'study' my responses. At that point I brought the mike up close and plunged in the dildo and orgasmed so big that it nearly knocked me unconscious. Afterwards I played it back, which made me come again, this time on my fingers so I could see how my contractions felt. This was my lesson!" Mrs. N. B. took advantage of a bit of voyeurism: "Being bisexual I have an advantage. I watched my girlfriend masturbate in front of me. As she was coming I felt all over her and learned about her responses in this way, because usually we come together and that's no good for serious study. It worked very well for my husband and therefore . . . keeps harmony at the hearth."

How do I fake? Depends on who I'm with and what I think they're looking for.

I stop breathing, like I'm holding my breath. I also open my mouth and let my head slip back. I don't have the energy for that thrashing business.

It's very simple. You breathe heavily, thrash around, moan intermittently, let out a big sigh: "Darling, you were wonderful."

I tense my stomach and let it ripple. That's what I do when I have a real orgasm.

Clutch, clutch. Make your pussy work. The joys of not having to display an erection!

Scream, shout and gouge his back. Gives him a memento. Gets rid of a bit of my frustration.

I am an actor by profession . . . and a very good faker.

The most famous Cecil B. DeMille of recent years appears in the film *When Harry Met Sally* (actually directed by Rob Reiner)— a marvelous concoction of groans, gasps, grunts, and gurgles.

Does Faking Mean She Hasn't Enjoyed the Sex?

No, no, no! Susan Quilliam reports that 57 percent of her sample of modern British women have faked. She also reports that 91 percent enjoy the sex. There are a myriad different reasons why we may find it difficult to have an orgasm on a particular day: pain, too much booze, tension, interruption, inability to find a good rhythm, no reason at all, or orgasm-killing comments such as "*I'll* make you come, my little pussy willow." Bella speaks for thousands of women:

There have been times when I've still been aroused but pretended to have an orgasm so that he would stop because I was afraid that the man was getting tired or bored with the whole thing, and I was afraid I wouldn't be able to have an orgasm no matter how long he tried anyway.

Putting an end to bad sex is only one reason among many.

Now imagine the following situation. You go to an exotic country south of the equator, get bitten by a poisonous puffer fish, and contract a mysterious disease. After a week of spots and fever, you find that in place of your once virile member you now have an anesthetized flagpole between your legs, erect but numb. The plus side, of course, is that your affliction quickly becomes the gossip of the day and ladies flock to your door to bounce and wriggle on your wonderful appendage for two hours at a time, before returning home to their husbands in a state of blissful exhaustion. But the minus side is serious. You now find it enormously difficult to climax yourself. Only with the greatest concentration can you work up the tiny sensations from your penis into an orgasm. Furthermore, it is like balancing cards. If your concentration is diverted before you come, you have to start building up the sensations all over again. But if you don't climax, the women are disappointed. They often take it as a personal insult, as if you're saying, "You're not pretty enough to satisfy me," and start to cry. One—a hulking great gym mistress—turns nasty and growls at you. Another is so determined to triumph over all her friends that she keeps you at it nonstop for five hours. By the end of the year your penis is too bruised to continue. You go to the hospital and have it chopped off.

How much simpler if you'd employed a little deception! If, on those occasions when climax was out of the question, you enjoyed sex for as long as you wanted, then writhed around and pretended that you'd come, everyone would be as happy as the circumstances allowed, and you could get back to work. Surely, you'd be a fool not to do it?

This is a good approximation of how it is for women on some nights. We fake when a real orgasm is out of reach. We don't do it for a laugh, very few of us do it all the time, and usually it's dependent upon circumstance: "Whenever I have had intercourse without any simultaneous clitoral work and I feel a duty (terrible isn't it?) to come, then I fake. Generally halfway through I'll decide whether to fake or not and I always congratulate myself on my performance."

So, if you discover that your lover has been faking, don't assume that all that furtive memorizing of *The Lover's Guide* has gone to waste and run off to join gay liberation.

This is not to say that bad sex isn't *also* a significant cause of faked orgasms:

> When sex is frightful, yet you like the guy, what can you do? Of course you can't say, "Excuse me, you are simply terrible." And if he's beyond redemption the only thing to do is fake yourself and then wiggle like crazy to make him come as soon as possible.

Did I Do Something to Encourage Her to Fake?

You are a man. Your very existence is encouragement for her to fake. Why? Because women know all about men's sensitive egos. One of the main reasons women cite for faking is entirely altruistic: to boost the man's self-esteem. "I fake to make him feel good" is a typical remark: "Wow, what a lover!"

> Yes, yes, yes!! I fake orgasms frequently. It fools him every time, makes him happy and makes him feel macho-like. I just breathe heavy, I shake a little, and tighten up my PC muscles and flex them. And you've got a man who thinks he's satisfied you.

So as not to upset his ego. It's easier—if much less sat-isfying—than having to explain things I don't really know myself.

I don't want to hurt his feelings, so I go to the bathroom and finish off.

I fake to make him feel good because he gets very wor-ried he may not satisfy me, but even when I don't or-gasm I am satisfied and he doesn't understand how that can be.

I faked orgasm because I did not want to hurt my image or my husband's. As a young wife I was supposed to be very sexual, ready to fulfill my husband's needs (in order for me to retain him at home). I wanted him to think that I was indeed "hot." You know the saying "lady in society, whore in bed." On the other hand I wanted him to feel he was "a good lover."

Women also fake to protect themselves; to spare what they see as their own humiliation. "Men *say* they want you to be honest, but they don't. They *hate* it. And of course it then re-bounds on you. You can't win." If you don't want her to fake, refrain from comments like, "My last girlfriend always managed it. I don't know what's the matter with you." Putting pressure on her is likely to drive her to deception, no matter whether you do it out of genuine desire to see her satisfied, or for rea-sons of vanity. As one lady succinctly commented: "Yes, I fake. Why? To get guys to stop pestering me about why not." What else can she do if she wants the sex to end pleasantly and with-out recrimination? True, most men don't turn nasty, but a dis-tressingly high proportion of women have had remarks of the "You're frigid" nature thrown at them, and it's not always pre-dictable who they'll come from.

I have only ever once faked an orgasm and I did it then because I was feeling inadequate and didn't want my partner to think there was something wrong with me. It didn't make me feel good to do it.

In my early twenties I faked it but soon realized it didn't matter since none of the men seemed to care if I did or not, so I stopped faking it. I didn't have my first real one until I was almost thirty. I used to fake it because I felt it made me seem more sexy and it would make him think he was a great lover. It seems like most (not all) black men feel very nervous if a woman has orgasm or enjoys sex too much. I always felt that it was my problem to deal with and I did not want them to think something was wrong with me.

With this partner most of the time I do fake it. Why? Mainly because if he thinks I didn't get off, I get an "I'm sorry" routine that reminds me of a child trying to get back into its parents' good graces.

On the days when I couldn't have an orgasm I felt like I did something wrong. Not move right or just not sexy enough. I would usually turn over, tell him it was great, then cry myself to sleep very quietly.

It saddens me that many women fake because they fear they will lose their man otherwise. "I have to fake to show I'm a great lover. If he knew I didn't come he might leave me for a better lover." In other words, being a good lover depends not only on what she does to the man, but also on having the correct responses herself. The burdens some people carry!

Often faking stems from sheer necessity: when you're raw inside, when dinner's boiling over, or when you feel a yeast infection or cystitis coming on. Why not tell the truth? Why not tell him about the cystitis for example? Because in the heat of passion it's a pretty unsexy interlude. He'll feel a little put off. She wants him to go ahead and enjoy his orgasm, but not to take too long. If she stops and explains about her condition, he's lost his momentum: this means an extra five minutes of painful bladder for her. *Plus* he's a decent guy and he'll probably feel he ought to withdraw immediately. She then says, "No, no, really it's okay to finish off." So he goes on, but feeling guilty now, not fully enjoying it . . . Some men actually *prefer* the odd "tactful" fake.

What Should You Do if You Suspect She's Been Faking?

Nothing dramatic. Spend the next ten minutes rereading this chapter and calm down. If you are really tormented with agony, ask—but not like this:

(*Scene: A bedroom. Harold and Jane lying side by side in bed, smoking. Outside, streetlights and the sound of traffic.*)

Harold: Aaah-em, Ja-ane?

Jane: Ye-es?

Harold: You awake?

Jane (*who is a suspicious type*): Why? What's up?

Harold: Nothing. I just wanted to, you know, as it were . . .

Jane: No, I don't know.

Harold: I don't know quite how to put this. I mean, I don't want to make you think I'm accusing you or anything, but . . . um . . . and I think our relationship should be open, don't you? I mean, honesty is the basis of love, don't you think?

Jane: Go on.

Harold: As I was saying, honesty is the basis of love and there is no truth without honesty, you wouldn't deny that, would you? No. Well, see, that's my point.

Jane: What point?

Harold (*sitting up suddenly and throwing his cigarette away*): You faked that orgasm didn't you? I know you did! Don't deny it! Why? Why? Why?

(*In the ensuing argument, Harold's cigarette butt sets fire to the curtains and the house is burned to the ground.*)

Everything is wrong here. The bumbling around at the beginning immediately puts Jane on the defensive, while the things said during the bumbling make it quite clear that Harold's feeling put-upon and accusatory. He's not trying to improve their relationship; he's introducing an air of moral blackmail. The final outburst—dreadful. Such tactics will never do.

The correct approach is to discuss the issue from the point of view of your improvement as a lover. In the house next door to Jane and Harold, Mr. Lincoln tackles the subject with considerable profit, while the sex is still going on:

Mr. Lincoln: You must tell me what to do. Men are such fools about women you know.

Mrs. Brown: Well, what you're doing with that finger does hurt a little. Move it an inch to the left.

Mr. Lincoln (*covering up his surprise. He'd always imagined she loved it where it was*): Like this?

Mrs. Brown: Much better. Now don't move in and out quite so much.

(*Pause*)

Mrs. Brown: Ahh! Oooh! Lovely! Eeek! Mmmmmmmm.

(*Pause*)

Mrs. Brown: I can smell burning. I wonder where it's coming from.

Faking has not come up, either in word or by suggestion. All the pressure is taken off her and transformed into a willingness to learn. If Mrs. Brown has not been satisfied this time, Mr. Lincoln can at least be comfortable in the knowledge that she considers him a first-rate lover.

Never *assume* she's faked: you can't possibly know, unless you've been a jerk and read her diary. *Remember* the axiom: No Woman Wants to Fake an Orgasm. Ask her what you can do to help, and make it clear that you don't mind. Encourage her to tell you when she doesn't want sex to go on any longer, and point out that for you, as a man, it doesn't matter because climaxing is easy.

The one type of faking that is really pointless, and which I disapprove of thoroughly, is doing it when the man's lovemaking is consistently wrong. Why encourage mistakes? If you suspect that this might be the problem, concentrate on giving as much pleasure as you can, in the least oppressive way. Don't impose your particular brand of sex on her just because it worked for another partner. Don't put pressure on her to perform. Do have plenty of room for discussion and improvement.

Otherwise, if she fakes now and then, it's no more important than the many little white lies we tell each other regularly. You know the sort of thing: she's just spent $50 on a new hairdo for a party. It's very fashionable, but you think she resembles a wedding cake. "How do I look?" she says, getting excited about the evening ahead. You grin and fake it: "Beautiful, darling." You refrain from ruining her evening, and resolve tactfully to dissuade her from another such disaster later.

Faking Can Be Good for You!

> I fake frequently because I know it satisfies my partner. He can relax if he knows I am enjoying myself. It also helps me loosen my inhibitions. If I can act wild, why not enjoy myself?

There are occasions when faking is positively recommended as a means to relax.

I used to suffer agonies of embarrassment about revealing to my partner that I'd never climaxed. Before I learned how to come during intercourse I was extremely ashamed that I couldn't do what most of the women in the world seemed to achieve effortlessly. I didn't fake for the simple reason that it never occurred to me. I loved sex and got highly aroused, but I felt I had to "come clean" at the outset and confess my "failing" in order to prevent worse awkwardness later on. This, however, often brought forth an "I'll make you come" response—the one phrase in the language designed to ensure just the opposite. It was doubly embarrassing when—lo and behold—he eventually discovered that he *hadn't* been able to live up to his boast.

One day I had the bright idea of faking—and never looked back. Instead of feeling tense and inadequate throughout sex I felt confident and in control. I thoroughly enjoyed myself. Because he assumed that I was able to climax there was no awkwardness between us; he didn't feel he'd failed or that he had to put on an extra special performance. Faking allowed me to concentrate on enjoying myself. And within a short time I had my first orgasm. Faking can be a very useful means to a successful end.

Nonfakers

Women who refuse to fake divide into two types: first, those who refuse to lie to boost a man's ego: "Fake? *Never!!* Why should I make him feel like he's accomplished something when he hasn't, and I like him knowing he's not up to snuff." Second, those who do not wish to compromise their own honesty. Carol writes, "I always feel crummy when I fake an orgasm . . . then my feeling crummy spills over into other things—compounding the error." One lady remarked simply, "I never fake. The truth is easier to remember."

There are those who have no theoretical aversion to it, but do not fake with their spouse because, "I've never climaxed and if I did he'd have candles and champagne to celebrate."

Certainly a relationship in which no faking is ever necessary would be most women's ideal, and one feels very keenly for Lynette, who, after years of lousy treatment from men, has the vigor to come clean:

> I fake it all the time. It's actually become a game to me now. I'm so good at it and it gives me a twisted sense of pleasure to know I can fool a man into believing he's a fantastic lover when he isn't. I know something he doesn't and I like that. In some sadistic way it's like a weapon, I can hurt him with the truth if I want or need to.

Not all men are nonfakers, it should be pointed out. Surveys show that a surprisingly high proportion of men have feigned orgasm, and that women are just as easily fooled in this respect. In *How to Have an Orgasm* I explained to women how to fake successfully, so it seems only fair to give men a little advice on this point as well. The fact that you haven't ejaculated inside her is, curiously, less of a giveaway than you might expect, because semen is unpredictable stuff. I've never understood why it is that some days after intercourse it comes gushing down immediately and soaks the bedsheets, and on other occasions you see no evidence until the next day. You set off beautifully dressed to meet the First Lady, and around four in the afternoon feel that ominous trickle between the legs. Naturally, this point doesn't apply if you wear a condom.

The main trouble for a man is his erection. If your penis usually goes limp very quickly after ejaculation, then she's going to wonder why it hasn't suddenly done so this time. So withdraw quickly or, if the matter comes up, point out that penises, just like everything to do with women's sexual responses, can vary greatly from day to day. As for the act, don't work it up too quickly, don't overplay it, and make sure you contract your penis rhythmically—about once every second, five or six times, with diminishing force toward the end—at the moment itself. This is what happens during ejaculation, when the semen is propelled into the outside world.

If your partner is suspicious, the semen smell (or, rather, the absence of it) is the most likely thing that will give you away. But she'll notice only if she's being very particular. Otherwise you're home and dry (hee-hee).

11

Orgasm: Women's Practical Advice to Men

*N*ot all women have difficulty climaxing. Those who don't will obviously have their own ideas about what is right for them. However, there are a number of sexual secrets that men can learn, and that may make all the difference between breathless satisfaction and stony-faced disappointment for women who have difficulty climaxing. Indeed, many can climax with ease providing the lover makes use of these skills.

Never call a woman cold because she doesn't climax with you. Don't even hint at it: it's old-fashioned, inaccurate, and cheap. She'll feel unpleasant, defeated, and under attack: everything will immediately be ten times harder. What's more, it's a completely misplaced remark. The inability to have an orgasm usually has nothing to do with not feeling aroused.

"I was *burning up* with unsatisfied desire," one woman fumed to me, "and he says I'm *frigid*!" It may well be that she had six wild orgasms with her previous man, in which case unpleasant accusations will simply rebound on your technique.

Do Not Put Pressure on a Woman to Climax

A very important and rarely heeded rule. It is even more important than your staying power because a sense of pressure can begin long before you get into bed and it conditions her frame of mind for the whole evening. Pressure kills desire stone dead. The most pernicious kinds of pressure are remarks along the lines of . . .

1. "I'll make you come, baby . . ." Any kind of promise or guarantee that you will give her an orgasm is not only strictly forbidden, it is suicidally foolish.

"Dah-ling," whispers the offender. "You'll scream with pleasure in five minutes flat once *I* get going."

Sheepishly Miss Darling protests that actually she hasn't been able to climax before, even though her last boyfriend was kind, caring, and well hung. The present lover dismisses three years of her life with a wave of his hand—"Just gimme five minutes and I will drive you *wild.*"

Miss Darling climbs dutifully into bed and waits for him to begin. He sets to work. He has said how she ought to react and therefore, feeling like a puppet in an X-rated Punch and Judy show, she can't manage to react at all. The whole night is set to become an appalling embarrassment.

Women hate this sort of approach to sex, especially from a new lover. A couple who have been happy and relaxed together for some time, and know what pleases each other, can just about get away with such promises. Even then it's risky. Many women have remarked how much they dread it when their husband guarantees he'll "give 'em something to remember," feel bad when he doesn't come anywhere close, and tense the next time around.

When a man talks to me about making me come, etc.—

I get turned off by that man and don't want to have any sexual relations with him.

2. "Let me give you some advice . . ." Having promised to make her scream with delicious joy in record-breaking time, and then failing to come anywhere close, the evil fiend now starts to give her the benefit of his wisdom. "You're too tense," he says. Or: "You know that you have to use your clitoris, don't you? You must stop thinking it's all in the vagina." Such educational remarks *might* have improved matters a hundred years ago when women thought sex was a question on census forms to which one appended the letter F or M. But nowadays, when we all happily masturbate?

> He was always saying, "You are trying too hard," or, "There is something wrong with you," or "You aren't relaxed enough" even though he was a sorry lover with a small penis.

The self-appointed orgasm oracle is a menace. A man never knows a woman's body better than she does, though many persist in thinking that they do.

3. "Everybody else has been satisfied . . ." Another howler. Where promises were egotistic, this is cowardly. It is Ex-girl-friend Man's stomping ground, and once again poor Miss Darling's hopes of orgasm are about to be thwarted. After going through all the preliminary stages with fitting expertise, the man suddenly pops his head up and says, in a tone of overdone surprise:

"No orgasm?"

She shakes her head, and thinks: "It's only been ten minutes. I'm not a water fountain."

"My ex-girlfriend used to come in five minutes."

Miss Darling's arousal level curls up and dies.

"All the other girls I've known could always come," he persists. "Am I doing something wrong?"

"No."

"Then it must be your fault!"

Such people are the scourge of the orgasm world and most women have met at least one:

> The famous "Everyone else has been able to" quote! And always the indignant "Why not?" I have never been able to turn around and say, "Because you weren't good enough." But I will one day.

There are a host of other unpleasant remarks in this category: Louise was deeply hurt when a man, having failed to "make her come" remarked, "Boy, you're a hard nut to crack."

> A man I'm with asks me if I've had an orgasm. If the answer's yes, I smile joyously. If no I feel guilty. I feel I'm taking too long, he's getting as anxious and frustrated as/with (me) not being able to get me there . . . I hate to feel the slightest bit of pressure. It makes my mind start saying it's not going to happen for me, he's been at it long enough. Just let him finish so that one of us gets satisfied. And it will cease the pressure of performance.

An insensitive remark can cause trouble for months or even years to come. Lulu describes herself as a blond American, twenty years old, married to a man more than twice her age who, as she points out, should have known better. For a long time sex was good, even though she didn't climax. Then one day, just after they'd made love, he started telling her in detail about how readily his ex-wife had orgasms:

> I took this very badly, because my interpretation was

that she was an excellent lover . . . I have very ill feelings about her to say the least—I consider her to be white trash. My feelings were deeply hurt because he had continuously been making a big deal out of something that had never come up in any other relationship I had been in . . . My husband made me feel terrible about myself, threatened, self-conscious and insecure . . . I usually never mind about not having an orgasm. I had never had any complaints before my husband, and when he mentions me not having one I mind immensely. It is almost like creating a sex phobia—I don't want to do it with him because I consider myself a failure.

It is extremely easy *not* to put pressure on your partner: banish the word "orgasm" from your vocabulary. As soon as you suggest that the main thing worth going for in sex is the ten-second wallop at the end of it, you're manufacturing trouble for yourself. Make it clear that you enjoy the buildup just as much and want to savor it to its full. Follow Susie's advice:

There's one big uniting characteristic about all the best lovers I've had—they make it clear they like sex. I don't mean they like orgasms. I mean they like all of it: foreplay, intimacy, relaxed intercourse. All of it. They like to make it go on pleasantly, like a really good conversation. With the best lovers it's like we're old friends messing around. Orgasm is just one part.

If *she* mentions orgasm, apply the same principle. Treat the subject lightly, not least because the woman's satisfaction can be a great burden to you as well if it becomes too much of an issue. Read up about the subject. The more you understand how women vary, the better you'll be able to satisfy her. *How to Have an Orgasm* is chock full of tips and advice.

If You Don't Know, Ask

The man who asks what a woman likes in bed is immediately elevated above the norm. If he does it properly, he's halfway to sexual stardom. But there's asking and there's asking. The crude method is rarely the most productive:

> **He** (*reading, over breakfast, this book*): It says here I should ask you what you want me to do in bed. I assume it will be a complicated answer. Could you write it down, so that I can memorize the solution in my spare time?

Sex and breakfast cereals do not go together. She feels like a fool and does not reply. *If* the question is to be asked in words it is best accompanied by gestures, while making love. In an aroused, receptive state, words can be kept to a minimum. Even a raised eyebrow, Roger Moore style, may be sufficient to imply "Is this okay?" Or you can be more forthright.

"What would you like me to do next?" whispers the sophisticate. "Tell me . . . tell me . . ."

Robert, a stocky, good-looking man who has spent his life traveling around the globe sweet-talking his way into one job or another, was nevertheless simply too embarrassed to ask his girlfriend what she wanted in bed, so he devised a rather cunning tactic:

> We were sitting up over a glass of tequila one night, drinking it with limes and salt on the back of the hand, and getting pretty in the mood, and we started to talk about sexual fantasy. I suggested that I be her sex slave, and she the cruel mistress. My sole purpose was to satisfy her in whatever way she ordered me to do. It was very enlightening . . . I learned things I could never

have asked. She guided my hand to *exactly* the right spot, and because of the fantasy it was easy for her to "chastise" me when I got it wrong. Best of all, it was my turn next . . .

Finding out what a woman wants during sex is not always easy, because she often won't speak up. There are a number of possible reasons for this: embarrassment, modesty, or (most likely) fear that it makes her sound selfish. Even quite strong, independent-minded women with partners longing to oblige their filthy desires may feel they shouldn't be "pushy" in bed. "I have a friend," writes Kirsty, "who can make herself come in twenty seconds, she masturbates everywhere and has no qualms about discussing it with us, but she does say that she is still shy about discussing sexual preferences with her partner."

Or a woman's silence may be due to simple uncertainty. Sometimes a woman just doesn't know what she likes best. Until you actually begin moving over her body, she can't say how she's going to respond. So when asking her directly doesn't get the information you're after, alternative measures must be adopted:

1. Listen to suggestive noises: Mmmmmmms and Aaaahhhhs can usually reliably be interpreted as "Yes, please continue." Pay careful attention to where she guides your hand: if she slides it gently to the left don't be obtuse and slide it back again to where it was! The boor Cheryl encountered is not a good man to imitate:

> I remember having a relationship with one man and trying desperately to get him to do the things I liked as gently and tactfully as I could with little Ums and Arrs. Yes, there. No, not there, etc. He suddenly stood up and said, "What are we doing, writing a book!" I felt ashamed but later very angry.

Of course, silence does not necessarily mean dislike. A woman might have put all her concentration into enjoying what you're doing, and have none left over for the encouraging murmurs. Or she may be one of those who goes mute and pale during her orgasm. In such cases, you must . . .

2. Listen to her body: Trembles, wriggles, tensing of muscles—they all signify something. Most of the time it will be obvious. When it's not, ask gently. If you suspect that what you're doing may be unwelcome, try suggesting: "Is this too ticklish?" which gives her a chance to put a stop to it with minimum awkwardness for both of you. Deep breathing is a good indication of pleasure and relaxation. Slow, rhythmic movement of the hips is another sign. If she suddenly bucks sharply and squirms like mad it's unlikely to mean you've touched the secret of feminine joy. More probably, you've hurt her.

3. Theatricality: A useful tactic for eliciting information and the stock-in-trade of sophisticated lovers. Suppose you suspect that sex is going on longer than she enjoys it—penetration, in particular. The trick is to suggest you're very close to climaxing by, for example, murmuring softly, "I can't last much longer." If she moans (apparently in ecstasy), "Oh darling, come inside me, yes, yes, yes" or words to that effect, it's because she's had enough. If, on the other hand, she immediately stops moving and says, "No! Wait! Think about dirty laundry," then you know she wants more. Once lovers get to know each other well they become adept at such ploys.

Knowing when to stop is the ultimate skill of the sophisticated lover. Not only is he prepared to keep going for a long time, he also knows when a long time turns into too long. It's a tricky one to learn, and instinct plays a part. If she does things obviously to excite you, such as varying the speed, or some sort of fiddling that you especially like, this too could be a sign that she wants you to bring the matter to your blissful conclusion.

It's fair to say that a woman is always alert to her man's responses, but men are often too wrapped up in their own sexual pleasure to notice the way the woman is reacting. The good lover must not fall into this temptation.

> In my marriage of twenty-two years my husband was body shy, bedroom shy and vocally shy—made up for of course in many other ways, but unfortunately the marriage finally and inevitably ended from lack of sexual activity. In the year and a half with my boyfriend, I learned a lot about talking. That helps the most, to openly and frankly state your preference. Of course at first I was too embarrassed to speak up. He would ask me what he could do to make sex better. What did I like or dislike? At first I couldn't tell him. I said: I don't know, I like it all, I guess? As time went on and being vocal about things was accepted and encouraged I was able to talk about such things as rhythm (his fast, mine slow), how to tilt my clit slightly up and apply pressure and motion to get a better climax for me, hearing words of sex was exciting, role playing was very interesting. A good-smelling man, nice body to look at. If all my senses are involved favorably the climax is more assured. That's taste, touch, smell, sight and sounds along with sincerity, wow! What a delicious combo! If I go back to my husband maybe my new behavior will help us learn more together.

Keep Going

The most common reason why women fail to climax is that men come too soon. A desirable lover is one who stays the course. Chapter 12 is entirely devoted to techniques men can learn to enable them to keep going for as long as necessary. Here I shall discuss it from the woman's point of view.

Most women need at least fifteen minutes, preferably longer. Since I devised my orgasm plan in *How to Have an Orgasm* I've gotten pretty good at climaxing, yet still there are days when I take ten minutes and days when I take forty-five. Bernard Zilbergeld remarks, in his otherwise excellent book *Men and Sex,* that if a woman doesn't have an orgasm in fifteen minutes, then the chances of her coming at all are "highly improbable." This is nonsense, and I have a pile of letters groin deep to prove it. The buildup to orgasm can be very slow and gradual:

> It is so different all the time. It depends on lots of factors. I come almost every time I have sex but sometimes it will take me next to no time, which is oddly quite often those times when I'm *not* feeling all that eager. Then there are also times when it will take half an hour. I can't make sense of it.

> I usually need about twenty to twenty-five minutes.

> The shortest was, I guess, two minutes. That was unusual. The longest (with the same man) was about an hour and a half. If I still had him I'd hire him out to the housewives around here whenever the mortgage payments were due. Slow, unpushy, casual, gentle, relaxed. He'd taught himself to be like that. If he knew I didn't mind, I could make him come in thirty seconds.

Make it clear that you *enjoy* going on for a long time. It's not enough to say, "No, no, I don't mind." You need to suggest that you *prefer* lovemaking to last, that it's extremely sexy for you when it is drawn out and unhurried. The ace bed partner knows that a considerable number of women fail to climax *only* because they worry they are taking too long. This has happened to me many times, especially in the early days of a love affair. One worries that, after twenty minutes or so, the man is getting impatient or bored. Then it becomes circular: the more one worries, the longer it takes—the longer it takes, the more one worries. "I could shoot him when he says, 'Well, we started out the same time, baby,' " exclaims Becky.

A Good Rhythm

> We are reminded of the popular custom in Thuringia. There a couple will not marry until the boy and girl have sawn through a log together. If the rhythm of their movements agrees, the marriage takes place, otherwise the association is broken off.
> —DR. SOPHIE LAZARSFELD,
> *WOMEN'S EXPERIENCE OF THE MALE*

There you have it. Go out and find yourself a log. Rhythm is decisive. When a woman masturbates, she does so with a given rhythm, unless she's feeling so horny that any movement at all in the right place will do the job. During penetration, it's the same. "Get the right rhythm," she thinks to herself. "Then pray it doesn't stop too soon." Pay attention to her words and gestures. Telling you to slow down, clasping your behind and making it move with her, gripping you harder between her legs—these are all methods of making you fall into the correct pace.

Dilly, a thirty-nine-year-old, writes bodice-ripping-style romantic fiction under a pseudonym. She produced an excellent description of the rhythmic buildup to orgasm, which is, she is quick to point out, dramatically different from the sort of whiz-bang-crash climaxes her heroines have:

Imagine an enormous flight of steps—lots and lots of

very shallow steps leading up to a stately home or mansion. You are convalescent after an illness and cannot rush ahead. You have to walk up gradually, putting both feet on each step. It's a long flight and you establish a gentle rhythm, all the way up to the top. Slow but sure. That's what the buildup to orgasm is like. Each step is a penis thrust: some days you need lots of the same tempo. You're getting to the top gradually. Men have a way of stopping three steps from the end.

A few women like vigorous penetration:

I come easiest when the man thrusts into me very fast and hard for a long time with me on my knees doggy style. When he eats me I like him to open up my labia and pull back my clitoris foreskin and suck and flick his tongue back and forth on my clit. If he doesn't apply enough pressure I cannot come. Another thing is to get him behind and beside you and thrust very slowly and deeply as I masturbate myself into a very hot orgasm. I like him to pinch and lick on my nipples and suck on my neck and he has to be a good kisser.

Because men in the heat of passion tend naturally to move fast, such preferences are easy to communicate. Slowing guys down is much more of a problem for women. Therefore be receptive to her words and gestures: *really* slow down if she asks, and don't hot up again after ten seconds. *Feel* for the pressure and rhythm from her hips.

Allow Her to Concentrate

Concentration is a vital ingredient for women who have difficulty climaxing, yet it is often neglected by women themselves:

"I don't want to try so hard, to have to concentrate so much, to have to work at feeling sexy or staying 'in the moment.' (My thoughts seem to stray so easily.)" For millions of women orgasm does not happen magically—at least not often, and we need to savor the sexual stimulation *without distractions.*

First deal as best you can with outside distractions. Children are the world record-holders for messing up sex, closely followed by thin partition walls, nosy neighbors, squeaky doors, and in-laws coming up the front path. Women can't separate sex from daily life as easily as men can, perhaps because sex usually takes place in their daily environment. (Try luring her to your office after hours and screwing on the boss's mahogany desk: you may find she has multiple orgasms while you are anxiously looking over your shoulder.)

Good concentration is also local. It means that at some point during lovemaking she may have to forget about you and put all her attention onto herself. Stroking a man's balls is nice to begin with but ultimately distracting. Conventional sex manuals rarely understand this point: they gaily advocate doing this, that, and the other simultaneously and don't realize that while it's making the man come quicker, it's slowing her down. Kari offered this excellent advice: "I have realized it is very important to be able to tune out everything. A pillow over my face works sometimes." Having oral sex is so popular with women because the whole emphasis is on their pleasure. They do not feel they ought to fiddle with him, because he's not within reach.

A woman also needs to be able to focus on a limited number of sensations on her own body. A phenomenon that I have called the Disembodied Woman is a very important aspect of female sexuality. It occurs when, even though the woman feels overall that she is getting more and more aroused, she doesn't seem to be getting any closer to orgasm. "My level of enjoyment and excitement vary," remarks Patricia, of this sensation. "It just doesn't seem to travel to the parts I need it to."

During sex, many things come into play. Not only is the man thrusting his penis in and out, he may also be stimulating his lover's breasts, nuzzling her earlobes, etc. Yet, in the final lead-up to a woman's orgasm, these attentions can be distracting even though they increase her overall desire. Many women need, at least in the last few minutes, to focus their concentration on only his penis thrusts. Even when his ear-nibbling *heightens* their overall excitement, it can still lead them down the wrong path—the path *away* from orgasm. The reason is because it replaces that badly needed concentration on orgasm with a more diffuse sensual pleasure. As Sally explains, it's almost as if for some women there are

> two parts to me. On the one hand there's the orgasm. I may want to have one very much or I mightn't mind too badly, but whatever my desire for it I must either go full out for it alone or give up. I've got to get the timing right and the rhythm and so on. I've got to think only about the feeling in my groin. It's like coming up to a hurdle in the steeplechase: you've got to make sure you jump from the right foot at the right time with the right stride and so on. On the other hand, there are the general body pleasures. I can just lie back and enjoy the idea of sex, or the feel of his hand playing over me, or the intimacy of his kissing and affections—but if I do that I'm limiting my chances of coming. As if my friends who'd come to watch me jump the hurdle began an interesting conversation among themselves as I ran towards it.

Long concentration on one part of her body is often more effective than a little bit of everything. As another reader put it: "I have come quite close. The reason I don't is about the time I reach the edge he stops doing whatever it is he's doing and goes to another part of my body." The pick and mix approach to sex—a little bit of everything—is best confined to foreplay. Susan, from New Zealand, speaks for many, many women: "Being quite passive in the missionary position and concentrating on my pleasure is the only way I can ever come unaided." She also gives an excellent description of the diffuse sexual pleasure women experience, which doesn't necessarily lead straight to orgasm:

> I met a man, a Korean, tall, beautiful and so sweet and wonderful that I'm quite smitten. The sex has consisted mainly of him trying hard to please me and me just being so blown away by his beauty and grace that I can't get anywhere *near* orgasm.

New positions are also excellent concentration destroyers for women. Assume, unless otherwise instructed, that she's more likely to climax in one of the old familiars. Finding the right position is so important that I consider it in detail in chapter 7.

Many women have never climaxed only because they have never concentrated fully on themselves and their own pleasure. They fear it is selfish, even though the man finds it sexy when his partner is self-centered. Therefore always encourage her to believe that far from being selfish, watching her enjoy the pleasure you are giving her is highly arousing for you too. One lady explained that she likes to be "in total control, I set the stage, I call the shots. Here's my favorite method":

> I make my husband lie down on the bed naked. I light candles and turn on music. I usually wear this pink clingy nightgown with spaghetti straps that I find very sexy. He is not allowed to touch me until I tell him he can. I dance and touch myself and give him occasional peeks. Sometimes I get on my hands and knees, with my bottom facing him, and slowly raise the gown over

my butt. I may get very close to him then and spread the lips of my vagina apart and may move one of my fingers in and out of the hole. I get very lubricated when I do this and it drives him crazy. But then when we finally have intercourse, I can't have a damn orgasm.

I'd hate to deprive her husband of a single moment of such erotic dancing (and he'd be a saint if he lasted more than five minutes after that!) but this lady needs to attend to her own pleasure too. She's in control of the story line, but all the concentration is on arousing him. Perhaps they could agree that on alternate days *she* lies down naked and compliant and is wholly served by him. She would then have time to focus on her own sexual responses.

Don't Forget the Clitoris

Enormous numbers of women can't come by penetration alone. They need a bit of extra clitoral stimulation. This does not mean that sex is the less for it, or that you haven't proved up to the job; it's just the way she's made. It may be the way you're made too: it might, for example, have to do with the relative position of her clitoris and your pubic region, which rubs against her. Don't waste time feeling that sex this way isn't "real sex." Concentrate on what works.

I can only come when he's playing with me at the same time. I make him suck me first. He lies back and I push my pussy over his face. I like to imagine him there, forced to do this to me. Sometimes I'll forget and keep going until I come over him. But during intercourse he has to play with me. I'll suck and lick him if the lubrication's not enough and then gently lower myself onto him. I love the feeling of being impaled. He masturbates me while I ride him. I'll make his hand do it the way I want it. When he comes, I sometimes take his penis out and make it squirt between my legs. I like to use his shaft after that. The head's too sensitive. If I rest my cunt on his shaft and move gently . . . I have an orgasm and fall on top of him.

I've never had an orgasm without clitoral stimulation and I personally don't believe it's possible, although one of my partners once told me that a previous partner of his had.

I like a finger up my butt too, it feels like there's no escape, its coming from both ends.

I can have an orgasm without added clitoral stimulation but I have more orgasms when I do or when he does.

Clitoral is the way to go!

Extra clitoral stimulation during sex can be gotten either by the woman using her own hand or you using yours. The trouble, when the woman is straddling you, is knowing how to put your hand in the most comfortable, effective position. Several readers suggested that a man use "his thumb—I just get him to put it flat on his pubic bone, where I rub myself against it. He doesn't even have to move it, as I can move to get the best sensations."

If your partner has difficulty climaxing and doesn't already use extra clitoral stimulation, suggest she try it, or start doing it for her yourself. A bit of manual help combined with penetration is often only an intermediate stage before a woman learns to climax through penetration alone. The Starfish position (described in chapter 7) is an excellent position for this.

It's Never Too Late . . .

> Those who have not experienced orgasm should not give up trying. I was thirty-eight when I first did, and it was wholly unexpected. I had been resigned for years to the thought that I was one of those women who "don't orgasm." Lack of relaxation or confidence, or a possible "mental block" can hinder or slow down though.
>
> —ELAINE, SHEFFIELD

It's never too late for a woman to learn how to have an orgasm. The length of time she has been without one has no bearing whatsoever on her likelihood in the future. Indeed, many women have success as they get older and more relaxed with themselves, and more confident. I have several letters from women in their fifties and sixties who found great and unexpected happiness (often after finally ending an old and stale relationship).

Orgasms constantly surprise women.

12

How to Keep Going . . .
For As Long As She Wants

Smiling, she chides in a kind murmuring noise,
And from her body wipes the clammy joys,
When, with a thousand kisses wandering o'er
My panting bosom, "Is there then no more?"
She cries. "All this to love and rapture's due;
Must we not pay a debt to pleasure too?"

—EARL OF ROCHESTER,
FROM "THE IMPERFECT ENJOYMENT"

*E*jaculating too soon is a disaster. There's no soft way to say
it. It's not a compliment to a woman's sexiness, or an embarrassment of riches, or a sign of your virility—all these excuses have been tried in an effort to buoy up the spirits of a
premature ejaculator, and none of them is any good. Something
has to be done about it before the relationship turns sour.

The good news is that something *can* be done, and that
something is fairly easy: a few basic tricks and a simple self-

training program. That's all. Even the fastest ejaculator can slow himself down to a very respectable length using these tactics.

First you must establish where *you* stand on the ejaculation speed scale. Look yourself up on the chart below in the left-hand column; gulp as you read your worth in the center column; get out the diary and start marking off the days when you reach the right-hand side.

What's the longest you can usually last?	Status	Amount of training to get to next stage	Steps needed
Less than 5 minutes	Very Bad	4 weeks–2 months	1, 2 & 3
5 to 10 minutes	Bad	3 weeks	1, 2 & 3
10 to 15 minutes	Middling	2 weeks	1, 2
15 to 30 minutes	Good	1 week	1
30 to 45 minutes	Very Good	A few days	1
45 minutes plus	Expert		

If you come out as "Bad" or "Very Bad," don't despair. Make yourself feel better with an evening at the bar telling the world what demanding hags all women are, but be sure to start the training program in the morning. In a short time you'll improve greatly. Every man can last as long as he wants, if he is prepared to do the training. But if you want the plan to work you must pick out your level *honestly*. If someone is looking over your shoulder at the moment, you can idly place your finger on the last line, nod in a suave fashion, and mutter, "What? Doesn't this column go any further? Tut, tut, some men!" But to yourself be true.

Clinical premature ejaculation is when a man has no control over his orgasm. It may occur within seconds or minutes, but once intercourse has begun he feels his penis rushing uncontrollably toward the crescendo and nothing short of immediate withdrawal and a cold shower will stop it getting there. In severe cases, he hardly has to touch his partner before it's all over. Not surprisingly, this condition can make a man unhappy and misogynistic, which in turn prevents him ever learning how to cure it. It can sometimes drive him to extremes of inventiveness, best practiced on wide-eyed young girls:

He: Oh, mmm, my gorgeous, you are so love-*phsst*-ly.

She: *Phsst?*

He: Afraid so. The end. Got a Kleenex?

She: But we've just begun, haven't we?

He (*inspiration dawns*): No, no. You're mistaken there. You fell asleep. We've been going on for ... ooh, an hour, minimum. Wore you out I guess, ha, ha.

The nonclinical type of premature ejaculator is predominantly selfish. He could last longer if he put his mind to it, but doesn't bother or hasn't yet realized that he ought to. His most distinctive characteristic is the habit of becoming hard of hearing the moment his penis starts to enlarge:

Man (*slotting in and setting to*): One, two, one, two, one, two.

Woman: Would you mind slowing down a bit?

Man: What's that, Sally? Oooh, aaah, mwooh.

Woman: Please slow down, plee-eeease, Bill.

Man: Mmmm, you're hot stuff, Sally. Quite a little nutcracker. Faster, faster, grr, grr, yum, yum—*phsst*.

We see here the basic difference between the clinical and the selfish premature ejaculator: if Bill had slowed down as asked (and women do frequently ask), he might have proved at least halfway satisfactory. As it is, Sally makes a mental note to avoid him next time: one bout of selfish pleasure has cost him an untold number of further sexual encounters. And yet, despite his sins, Bill's problem could be solved simply by reading Step One. It's a matter of just applying and polishing up the control he has hitherto neglected, and supplementing it with a few basic techniques.

The plan divides into three steps. Step One gives all the good tricks for delaying your climax, which can be implemented immediately. Steps Two and Three teach you how to develop full control over your climax.

STEP ONE:

Techniques to Adopt Immediately

Start with fiddling (i.e., foreplay)—plenty of it, in all its variety: it's the simplest and most common way to avoid an unequal ending. However, because it is often hard to gauge when a woman is close to climaxing, it's by no means a fail-safe approach. The change of rhythm and type of stimulation can mean that, although your partner was quite close to being satisfied by fiddling, she is still a good way from having an orgasm by intercourse. The only way to get around the problem completely is to make sure that she climaxes before you penetrate.

The Oriental Technique: A New Type of Thrust

Practiced for thousands of years, this is the most basic coital tactic and the most immediately successful. If you're already a ten-minute man, it will double your time at a stroke. Learn the technique properly and there will be, theoretically, no limit to your longevity. In one form or another it appears in all Eastern erotic books that deal with delaying ejaculation.

The rationale for adopting a new type of thrust during intercourse is to take advantage of the different way in which men and women get aroused: for the man it is by friction against the shaft of his penis, whereas for the woman it is due to friction, not inside her vagina, but against her clitoris, farther up. From this asymmetry spring glorious solutions, though few lovers exploit it properly. The best way to illustrate what I mean is by comparison.

Let's begin with Mr. Ordinary Thruster. He climbs into bed, inserts, then spends a certain amount of time rapidly moving his penis in and out. He does this in the conventional way by pulling his hips away from his partner and sinking back down again. Traditional though this technique is, Mr. Ordinary Thruster is putting most effort into arousing his own organ. The amount of excitement his partner gets to her clitoral region is limited to when he's fully inside, pubis to pubis. After ten minutes, she's had the equivalent of, say, a minute and a half of direct stimulation.

Mr. Thriller Thruster is much less vigorous. He inserts slowly and moves slowly. Instead of pulling himself away from the lady at every thrust, making a gap between them, he remains in close contact on top of her. Because of this abbreviated movement, his pubis, stomach, and upper thighs are constantly stimulating her instead of propelling him outward. He does not move so passionately, but he is a lot better at inducing passion in his friend. Looked at from above, the bodies seem to be on water, moving with the waves. By this simple adjustment, after ten minutes, *both* partners have had ten minutes of stimulation.

If Mr. Thriller Thruster starts to get too excited, he can calm his movements even more. He keeps his *penis* entirely still inside his partner, but continues to move his *hips* gently, thereby continuing to stimulate her, while keeping his own stimulation to a minimum. After ten minutes of this, he's had the equivalent of about three minutes, while she's had the full quota.

Rosalind is one of the many women who are happy to have intercourse almost entirely made up of this limited type of movement:

> Yes, yes! It's so obvious and so effective! He can pretty much keep still altogether if he needs to. I mean, for you it's still great. You've got his dick where you want it, and you've also got the pressure where you need it most. Okay, so he's not being a powerhouse, and sometimes that's what you really want, granted. With this technique you get a bit of in out, in out, but mostly it's a case of swirling it around and around, grinding, slowly, getting you worked up without the threat of each thrust about to make him pop.

There are a number of variations of the approach, which can be used according to mood:

The Glider: The basic technique. The man keeps his penis fully inside, and moves his hips gently over the woman's clitoral region. One of the attractions of this calm type of intercourse is that, in reducing the heated concentration on the genitals, it allows other things of a kissing and feeling nature to go on undistracted. It is very pleasant as a way to vary the pace of sex, and many women, like Rosalind, are quite happy if their partner uses this approach most or all of the time. To produce extra pressure, you have only to rest on your elbows, because this puts more weight on your hips.

The French Polisher: Best done with someone you know well or during playful sex—you're liable to end in giggles. The French polisher moves his hips in small circles over his partner's loins, taking care to make the focus of the pressure between her legs. It is not the most natural of movements and a man has to be quite supple in his lower back to keep it up for long. Nevertheless, it is good if done well. Zilbergeld relates the following:

> One man, almost legendary for this lengthy sexual encounters, shared his secret with us. Many years ago he considered himself to be a sexual flop because he came very quickly when he received any stimulation from a partner. He had no one from whom to get help, this being long before the advent of sex therapy, so he decided to experiment with different masturbation techniques. He discovered that by using a circular motion, employing the base of his penis as a fulcrum and moving the shaft and head in small circles, he had complete control of when he ejaculated. He then transferred his discovery to sex with partners. In intercourse, for example, instead of moving in and out of the vagina he inserted his penis as far as possible and, moving his hips in a circular motion, moved it around the vagina. When he wanted to come he started thrusting in and out. Both he and his partners were quite satisfied with the results.

Note the first sentences: from flop to legend by the simple expedient of changing the type of his thrust. Very accomplished French polishers like to alternate clockwise with counterclockwise movements or vary the speeds to suggest a tune, etc. Judge from your own circumstances whether you can get away with such modifications.

The Starfish: The Starfish position (described in chapter 7) proves its usefulness once again! Lying on your side with the woman on her back, you can use your thigh to press between her legs and excite the right parts, while moving your penis only minimally. She can hold on to your leg and change the angle and pressure to suit her taste. You both, meanwhile, can chat about the weather, who's going to do the dishes, or the un-

speakable things you'd like to do to each other on a desert island. The Starfish also allows the man to provide extra manual
stimulation, which will increase his partner's satisfaction even
more.

If, in spite of all, you still find yourself growing too heated,
then stop moving completely. Simple and effective. It will give
you time to get back in control. Louise:

> It turns me on when a man suddenly whispers "Stop!" in
> my ear. Like he's about to break down and fill me up. It
> gives me a real lurch. I hold him there and think about
> the semen that's almost at the top of his prick and the fact
> that he's nearly out of control. Then pretty soon he's mov-
> ing again, and I let go of my breath and start to reply until
> once more I've brought him near to collapse.

The one complicating factor is that your partner may not always appreciate how important it is for you to slow down or
stop. If you're feeling close to the critical moment, a burst of
passionate wiggles from her is the last thing you need.

How Do I Get Her to Understand That I've Got to Stop Moving?

1. Explain

2. Theatricals

3. Threat

4. Withdraw

1. Explaining is not the most romantic approach, but it is
straightforward. Announcing stolidly, "I'm about to come" is

quite unsexy. Saying, in a breathy, quivering way, "Please! Stop! You're driving me wild! I'll explode!" (or something similar) is more in the mood of the moment. Appealing to the vanity of your partner—in this case, her mind-bending eroticism—is always the best route forward. For experiment, it is worth pretending you're about to climax when you're not. Then you can study the way she reacts to the news and know how to conduct yourself in the future. Another occasion on which such pretense is useful is when you think she might have had enough. If you sense this, then tense your body, make the appropriate guttural noises, and say your I'm-getting-too-close-please-slow-down number. If she replies "Go on, drown me, baby" or similar, then the time is ripe. Do as she asks.

2. Theatricals are useful on those evenings when you find yourself irreparably oversensitive. It involves "pretending you're in a coma or have gone to sleep," explains Julian. "I say to Lilly: 'I'm terribly tired. Just pretend I'm asleep.' I lie on top and she moves. Because she's underneath she can't move all that much and because I'm not moving at all, it means that overall there's a lot less excitement down below." But with good positioning and gentle hip movement, the man can still ensure that his partner gets plenty of attention. With a bit of inventiveness, fantasies involving gravediggers, nurses, and anyone else likely to come in contact with the immobile and the comatose can be adapted to serve the same purpose.

3. Threat. Sometimes necessary with a woman who has gotten carried away. It is explanation without the artifice of number 1, as in: "I'm telling you. Stop. Else it's over and that's it for the night." This is a risky approach.

4. If things are really close, **withdraw** quickly. A minute's pause can put off your ejaculation for up to ten minutes. Because women cool off much less quickly than men, when you begin intercourse again your partner will have kept much more of her original level of arousal than you have. In the meantime, if you worry that she'll get bored hanging around waiting for you, you can keep up her interest by using your hand or your mouth.

The Pacific Technique: Pelvic Floor Exercises

Anthropologists have discovered several societies, such as the Marquesas islanders in the Pacific, where the men time their climax by using the muscles of the pelvic floor, otherwise known as the pubococcygeal, or PC, muscle. Learning how to use it for ejaculatory control depends on two things: developing its strength, and experimenting to discover what works for you. Some men find that once they've got good control of the muscle, they can stop ejaculation by relaxing it at a critical moment just beforehand; for others, tensing it is the key.

Since this subject is discussed in full detail in the next chapter, "How Men Can Teach Themselves to Have Multiple Orgasms," I won't say any more about it here.

Special Points to Press and Sundry Other Tips to Delay Ejaculation

Most of these are not very helpful, unfortunately, but they are worth trying.

Between the testicles and the anus, there exists an oft-forgotten region known as the perineum. By pressing here very firmly, it is possible not only to delay ejaculation, but to prevent it altogether. A Chinese erotic manual, *Classic of the Immortals,* advises, "When, during the sexual act, the man feels he is about to ejaculate, he must quickly and firmly press with fore and middle finger of the left hand the spot . . . simultaneously inhaling deeply and gnashing his teeth a score of times, without holding his breath."

The snag is that ejaculation and orgasm are not the same thing, hence the need for all that extra gnashing. By pressing this point, the man is blocking the flow of semen through the vas deferens as it comes from the testicles on its way to the penis. If he feels he's just on the point of climaxing, a quick gouge down there will simply stop the semen appearing, but it won't delay the orgasm any more than will gripping his penis very hard to close off the urethra. He'll still go quivery and, shortly after, limp.

The Secrets of Sexual Desire, a Sanskrit book from before the fourteenth century, claims that "if one at the time of sexual enjoyment presses firmly with the finger on the fore part of the testicle, turns his mind to other things, and holds his breath while doing so, a too rapid ejaculation of the sperm will be prevented." This sounds rather painful. I don't recommend it. A third point is said to be above the right nipple.

A last-resort way to get around the annoyance of premature ejaculation is to ensure that you have a quick snooze after climaxing. Men—especially young ones—are quite often fresh again after just a few minutes' sleep, whereas the same period awake would have made hardly any difference at all. So put the alarm on for a ten-minute slumber, and try again. Someone ought to do a Ph.D. thesis on the subject and revolutionize the world. What is it in the brain that is recharged or cleansed by sleep, even brief sleep, and that relates to sexual desire? And can pharmaceutical companies turn it into a sugar-coated tablet? No doubt, like all other good things in life these days, it has something to do with serotonin.

First-Night Nerves (Drastic Measures)

There are times in our sexual life when stern approaches must be adopted, and the first night with a gorgeous new partner is one of them. Plenty of foreplay and limited movement during intercourse may not be enough.

The most obvious device is the crudest: masturbate beforehand. It's not romantic, but she won't know and first nights are rarely subtle occasions. They're testing ground for the second and subsequent nights. Peter:

> On the times I've done it I've always felt a little disgusted with myself, especially directly afterwards, in the cold neon light of the disco toilet with my penis gone limp and my hand wet with come, when I can't imagine why I ever wanted to get involved in this sex business anyway. But then practicalities must be faced. I've got to prioritize: I've struck lucky. I'm with a gorgeous woman who wants to come home with me. If I want more than a coarse one-night stand—if I want romance to blossom and hearts to flutter and her not to kick me out of bed—then I must be prepared to do a little coarse work beforehand. Nothing is ever pure honey and roses.

Time it well! Too soon before the real thing, and you'll be limp as overcooked asparagus. Too long before, and the advantage will have worn off. Depending on your age, between half an hour (for the under-twenties) and two hours (over-forties) beforehand is the critical period.

Incidentally, women sometimes do the masturbation trick too, but for the opposite reason. While you go off to the bathroom to clean your teeth we whip out a sexy novel and excite ourselves as close as we can to orgasm to get a head start. I know someone who keeps a large dildo beneath the bed. She plies her men well with drink, which works two ways—it slows them down, and takes them off to the bathroom halfway through. Whereupon she summons up her dildo for a three-minute bout (the toilet is down a long corridor).

Another straightforward trick for the start of a new relationship is to use a thick condom. Your own pleasure is diminished, naturally, but it's worth the sacrifice. However, thick Durexes are getting hard to come by. Gone are the days when eighteenth-century gentlemen enveloped their members in sheep gut in order to protect them from the consequences of their lust. Chemists are getting cleverer and cleverer at making even the toughest material thin and sensitive. You may need two: or five if you're feeling uncontrollable. The novelist William Gerhardie used this approach for different reasons. On a visit to Algiers he made a tour of "the houses of ill-fame for which Algiers is ill-famed, but my instinct for self-preservation," he explained, "causes me, in this place, to multiply precautions so that I feel I might be in a padded overcoat."

Penis desensitizers can also be bought in the form of anesthetic creams and sprays. Look in the back of dirty magazines for the relevant advertisements. Booze serves the same function up to a point, not only physically but psychologically calming the nerves that make a man either impotent or premature. But bear in mind that alcohol has quite a strong dampening effect on most women's orgasms. Marijuana also works to delay ejaculation for some people. As a last resort, you can try the Michael Caine method of delay, described by Adam, a twenty-nine-year-old London accountant:

> I'd just been watching *The Ipcress File*. Michael Caine—resourceful guy. There's this part when the bad character (can't remember his name) is trying to brainwash Caine by putting him in a big box that jiggles and makes psychedelic pictures and sounds. But Caine manages to resist this by forcing a nail into his palm to focus his mind on reality. It works. So, thinks I, that's the solution. About to squirt? Squeeze a thumbtack. If

that doesn't take your mind off matters amorous, then nothing will.

Other drastic measures include thinking about dirty laundry, clicking your teeth together one thousand times, imagining yourself having to walk along a very narrow branch—they work in the same way that hiccup cures and magicians work, by distracting your attention from the real action.

If the worst comes to the worst and you do climax sooner than she wants, try simply keeping going. Force yourself. Reduce the movements down to a minimum, put maximum emphasis on what you do with your pubis, and slow down to a rhythmic crawl. But keep going. Even when you've gone limp you can still do a girl a lot of good. Turn to oral or manual sex if that's easier. It's a matter of mind against temporarily vanished libido and with a bit of willpower you can manage it. In half an hour you'll be pleased that you did.

STEP TWO:

Learning Control on Your Own

If you're one of those who has no control over his climax at all, the above techniques will not have much effect yet. You first have to learn the basics. Don't waste your money going to a psychologist who'll fill you up with nonsense about sex guilt. Premature ejaculation, however it originated, is cured by training. The process can take several months, and the skill may not be perfected for yet a longer period after, but *the method is sensible, gradual, and highly effective.*

The idea that a man can learn to control his orgasm was first put into practice by the divinely named James Semans in the 1950s.

Without realizing it, [writes Zilbergeld] you have already successfully negotiated a very similar training process: when you learned to control your urinary function. When you were very small, you had no control over urination; it just happened when your bladder reached a certain degree of fullness. But then your parents let you know that this was not satisfactory and that you had to take charge of the situation. You gradually learned to recognize the sensations in your body announcing that you were about to urinate, and you could signal that you had to go to the bathroom. At this point your training was incomplete. You could tell if something was about to happen but you couldn't delay its occurrence.

As time went on, you completed your training. You not only knew when urination was imminent but you could also exert some control over when it happened. You might realize that you had to urinate, but if you were in the middle of an interesting game you could squeeze some muscles and wiggle around enough to hold it back, at least for a while.

The Exercises

Find yourself a nice, quiet place where you're not going to be disturbed. I feel that it's better to embark on a self-help program of this nature alone. Involving your partner early on puts added pressure upon you to show results. But that is your choice. You will have to involve her in the next step anyway. The main worry about pursuing Step Two in secret is that she may discover you masturbating. A woman is often depressed by this, because she believes you're doing it to yourself because you don't like doing it to her. So be prepared with explanations, and have this book at hand. She'll be quite mollified when she learns you're privately teaching yourself to improve your performance for her benefit.

Each exercise should be practiced at least three times a week: the more the better.

1. Masturbate for fifteen minutes without ejaculating. If you feel yourself getting close to the point of no return, stop and calm down. When you're in control again, continue. Keep going until the fifteen minutes is up.

The object is not to bring yourself to the point of climax as many times as possible and then knock off just before it all spills out. The point is to learn how to govern your sexual response. Since most men masturbate at high speed, lasting for fifteen minutes will be difficult at first. So, pace your pleasure. Don't make your movements fast and furious. Once you've taught yourself to last the fifteen minutes with only two stops, go on to the next exercise. Keep track of your longest times.

2. Masturbate for fifteen minutes without ejaculating. If you feel yourself getting close to the point of no return, *instead of stopping,* change the way in which you are stimulating yourself so that it is less effective. For example, apply less pressure, or move more slowly, or rub over only a limited area, or think about slime and bogeymen. To begin with make sure your style changes quite significantly, so that your arousal diminishes and you have to resort to your earlier style to bring yourself back within sight of climax. As you get better at doing this, try to maintain a certain level of excitement for the whole of the quarter of an hour instead of chopping and changing.

3. The next exercise is to increase gradually the degree of arousal you can tolerate during masturbation, without ejaculating. Once you've mastered stage two, start to make the circumstances more exciting. The point, you must remember, is little by little to make these masturbation exercises approximate more and more closely the circumstances of intercourse. The closer you can get to the real thing while still controlling your orgasm, the easier you'll find it to keep that control with your lover. Steve:

> The simplest is to make the lubrication nicer. I found making it warmer also was good because it was more natural. It got me used to the pleasant feeling of warmth that usually just sends me crazy in a woman.

Another man tried a different technique. Just as the king's daughter in the French erotic classic *L'Ecole des Filles* had a bronze statue made with an erect, hollow phallus attached that discharged a warm liquid when she mounted it and touched a spring, Andrew, a mechanic . . .

> Jesus! I feel like I'm blushing just to think of it. Well, here goes: I made a doll. I was far too shy to buy one. I was convinced that if I sent off to one of those places in the back of porn mags that they'd forget to put the damn thing in a decent brown parcel. I could just see the postman knocking on the door and handing my wife a big package with "Pervert's Plaything" written in red letters on the top . . .
>
> I was certain that a doll was the best thing for it. You can't get much closer to life and still be alone than that, can you? If I could manage that, I was away. So I made my own. I won't go into details, except that it involved the comforter, a borrowed bra stuffed with socks, a roll of toilet paper with a plastic bag inside (that was the vagina) and plenty of warm water and shampoo for lubrication. It made the most terrible stain everywhere. But it worked for me. At first I could hardly hold at all, just like normal. With a bit of practice I got much better. My wife was delighted. I never told her how it came about though!

Another obvious way of making yourself better at control in more arousing circumstances is to watch a blue film or read a pornographic magazine while doing the exercises. Once again, if you get caught it's time for some delicate and fast explanation. First, show her this book and point out that you were acting under orders. Second, take the opportunity, since you will find no better one than this, to discuss your own worries about climaxing too soon, and warm her up to the idea of taking part in Step Two of your training. Use all the gentle arts: persuasion, reason, flattery, delicate self-criticism (but not so much as to depress yourself). Point out that the porn mag is there only because your imagination is too rotten to keep a decent fantasy going, then challenge her: "Do you mean to tell me you never have fantasies, even when you're doing it to yourself?" This, and similar Jesuitical techniques, will usually win the day. Best of all, get her to sit down and watch it with you. It's absolutely untrue that women don't respond to pornography. Many of us love it.

Whether you use videos, novels, or your own imagination, learn to control yourself for the fifteen minutes. If you find that the circumstances are too arousing, change them; eventually you will aim to make them as arousing as possible, and still control your climax. Do this exercise two or three times a week or more. Again, if you can, keep it going for longer than the quarter of an hour.

Once you've got to this stage, you're well on the way.

STEP THREE:

Learning Control with a Woman

Now it's time to bring in your partner: a big leap, since it is the presence of a woman that causes the difficulty in the first place. Nevertheless, the earlier exercises will have prepared you well. Keep them going while you continue through the ones that follow.

Getting your partner involved may seem embarrassing at first. However, women are usually understanding. We're always dieting and exercising, anti-celluliting, and waxing ourselves, so it probably won't seem odd at all that you want to do a bit of improving work on your penis. Besides, she's the one who's going to benefit. Just make sure you don't *neglect* her. Reread the "Fiddling" chapter if you're short of ideas.

4. Masturbation in front of your partner. This exercise is important because it represents a small progression from the first three exercises, but it also makes you more sexually relaxed with a woman. Discuss this with your partner first. Women often find it very sexy.

> I love it when Bill does it. It makes me really hot and it's new. I watch him and tell him when to stop and when to start. I get carried away sometimes and imagine that I'm a slave owner ordering my slave to humiliate himself in front of me. Whenever he gets close to coming I make him stop. Then I finally make him go all the way and insist that the semen goes on the floor (I usually make him do this in the kitchen where, fortunately, we have easy scrub tiles). After that I do it to myself and he watches.

> It's different. I also like it because it's cleaner and not so fussy. There's no stripping off and getting my panties dirty. I don't have to go to the toilet afterwards. He has to use the tissues. Then it's such a turn-on seeing him there in this totally vulnerable position. I mean, imagine if I took a photo of him then ran out and had it published!

> I once came home early from work and found Rupert lying on the bed jerking off. He went bright red. He tried to pretend he was doing something else and ram-

bled off some completely far-fetched explanation. I waited until he'd finished and said: "Get back on that bed and make yourself come. I want to see."

Keep going for a minimum of fifteen minutes, longer if possible. Fifteen minutes of masturbation alone is pretty boring; with a woman watching, things become distinctly interesting. A lot of men/couples who reached this stage were surprised to find how sexy indirect sex can be. If you feel silly or self-conscious, try having her sitting behind you, with her arms around you. Keep practicing this exercise until you feel quite sure of your control.

5. Now it's time to have contact with your partner, but the least intimate form of contact: ask her to perform manual sex on you. The object is to keep this contact up for as long as possible before climaxing. Before she starts actually rubbing, just play around for a while. Get used to having her there, near you, touching you, without feeling the urge to ejaculate. When she begins manual sex, have her keep it light and unhurried. Let her vary the pace and pressure, so that you don't start focusing too hard on the end result. Whenever you feel yourself getting too close, take time off to discuss what you're going to have for supper. If things get really hot have a chat about old socks and greasy pillowcases. When the passion has subsided and your self-control has returned, begin again. Be sensitive to what it is that makes you overheated, and learn to govern it. As Larry points out:

> It's the way she looks when she's doing it to me. There she is doing this thing, and looking as if butter wouldn't melt. I imagine her walking around afterwards and you'd never imagine that she'd just had her hands around me. I had to make her lie beside me at first. We were both on our backs, and she reached over and

used her hand without looking at me. We just sat there, chatting. After a few days, I got used to it, and she could move closer and take more part. Then she got so turned on, I had to make her climax beforehand. That was even better, because it meant I got used to keeping myself in over a really extended period, and didn't feel guilty or tense when I did come, which is one of the worst aspects of doing it too soon. You feel guilty and a disappointment. When next time comes around your head is going crazy with worry that you're going to be a disappointment again. You get yourself so tense and crazy that you sort of arouse yourself that way, so that you are a disappointment again.

6. Final exercise: penetration. Don't be in a hurry to get onto this. Like the last stage, it can be graduated in numerous ways. Begin by letting your penis move around between her legs and over the general area, but without penetration. Get used to the idea of being about to have intercourse without feeling the need to climax immediately. When you feel in full control, insert. The Starfish position (see chapter 7) is best for this. It is comfortable, without placing too much arousing concentration on you. The woman on top is also good, but less remote.

(a) The first and extremely important step of Exercise 6 is penetration without movement. Remain still—for the full fifteen minutes, if necessary—until you feel there's no risk of you climaxing. All the while you are getting used to her body—her warmth, moisture, and the abstract excitement of knowing yourself to be inside her. If you find your penis getting limp with the lack of movement, move a little—slowly and calmly. You should practice this exercise until you feel fully in control, no matter how long it takes.

(b) We come to the very last step: penetration with movement. Remember, you are not aiming to thrust away with a penis that is nigh on anesthetized. With vigorous thrusting, nearly every man will come too quickly because he is concentrating on massaging only the shaft of his member rather than stimulating his partner as well. Rather, you want to focus on slow, slight movements. Lie there with your hips moving, slipping in and out gently and not by much. Keep your mind on the fact that, to give your partner satisfaction, you want to make sure there is pressure from your pubis against hers. This will stimulate the clitoris. If you feel yourself losing control, stop. Withdraw.

It only remains for me to say again how highly appreciated is the man who can keep going. For women, worrying that their partner is going to come too soon is often the only hindrance to orgasm. Therefore, it is important that you establish that you can *always* last a good long time. Only then can she really relax and enjoy your passion.

13

How Men Can Teach Themselves to Have Multiple Orgasms

*T*eaching yourself to have multiple orgasms depends on recognizing a crucial fact that is almost always overlooked, even, until recently, in the scientific literature: ejaculation and orgasm are not the same thing. It is possible to have one without the other. Learn how to control your body so that you can separate them, and you will be on the way to having multiple orgasms. The process takes time and exercise, but the results are remarkable. So remarkable, in fact, that in 1984 Dr. William Hartman and Marilyn Fithian entitled their book on the subject *Any Man Can: The Revolutionary New Multiple-Orgasmic Technique for Every Loving Man*.

Any Man Can is a difficult book to get ahold of, despite its enticing title. The copy in the Cambridge University copyright library has been stolen. The British Library copy has also mysteriously disappeared. I eventually got ahold of this rare item in Oxford's Bodleian Library, photocopied what I needed, and then this too promptly disappeared into thin air! Suspicion fell on the garage man, the hotel maid, and a peculiar-looking waiter at the restaurant where I'd had supper. So I was obliged to make the long journey back to Oxford to get another photocopy, which I guard like a hawk. Every man I mention the book to begs to be allowed to borrow it. This chapter contains an improved, updated version of their remarkable program, together with all the important new information on this revolutionary subject that has appeared in the last decade. It has worked wonders. Hartman and Fithian, who helped to found the Center for Marital and Sexual Studies, California, in the 1960s, taught all sorts of men how to become multiorgasmic, including one who was impotent and another who was so severely handicapped that he was "totally confined to a wheelchair . . . easily fatigued, had trouble breathing, often had pneumonia, and had a tracheotomy in his throat, to which his respirator . . . could be attached." Nevertheless, he followed the program and it worked. "He and his partner came in, let us 'wire' them to our machines, and proceeded to make love. As he had predicted, they both had multiple orgasms. Yet he had to use his oxygen tank to keep from tiring."

The Different Types of Multiple Orgasm in Men

Men who have multiple orgasms can be divided into three types: those who have always had them, those who suddenly start to have them without doing anything to encourage it, and those who teach themselves how to have them. The novelist D. H. Lawrence (though he lost the knack in later life and became impotent) belonged to the first type. One of his early mistresses, Alice Dix, remarked that he "did come back to a woman time after time," and several of his novels have characters who are multiorgasmic as young men. Men who have the gift naturally are always surprised when they find out they're unusual. It's usually a delighted girlfriend who first tells them that they are not the norm.

Men who become multiorgasmic naturally often do so in their thirties, after considerable sexual experience. It happens by surprise and, when questioned about it, they can offer no explanation. Drag them into a laboratory, however, and an interesting thing can be seen. The first orgasms are almost always without ejaculation. The final orgasm, after which the man feels he cannot go on any further, is accompanied by ejaculation. The more the man can delay the ejaculation, the more climaxes he can have. The first scientific study of the subject, in 1978, found that although one man could have up to thirty in an hour, most manage between three and ten during one session of intercourse. They all agree that it's best when they're in a close, loving, stable relationship with a woman who is sexually cooperative.

The men who have *taught* themselves how to have multiple orgasms do it by taking advantage of this difference between dry and ejaculatory ones. They develop the muscles in their groin so that they can prevent the external sphincter of the bladder letting through seminal fluid during a climax. In normal circumstances, this sphincter relaxes involuntarily, allowing semen to flow from the seminal vesicle (where it's made) into the urethra and on up and out. The trick is therefore to gain voluntary control over the region. Some researchers have suggested that multiorgasmic women use the same approach with the corresponding parts of their bodies, though it's usually done involuntarily.

The physiology of orgasm, single or multiple, is still not properly understood, in men or women. Although the above explanation seems the most likely one, there are all sorts of oddities that any man who is interested in improving his performance can experiment with. It is notable, for example, that simply holding your penis very firmly during orgasm to prevent the semen coming out doesn't work. Pressing the perineum firmly (see chapter 12) is not usually successful either: it stops the semen from flowing up the penis, but it's too late from the orgasm point of view. Something inside has already registered that ejaculation is taking place and so multiple orgasm is not possible. On the other hand, some men do have multiple orgasms with a small ejaculation each time. Others ejaculate the first time, and then go on to have a host of further dry orgasms. "With a bit of willpower," says Terry, thirty-nine, "a man can also do this: have an ejaculation without an orgasm, and then have the orgasm later. You have to concentrate extremely hard at the time and force yourself not to react when you ejaculate. You mustn't let the tiniest sensation of orgasm escape. Just relax totally and resist. Wait till the semen's out and then keep going. It's debatable if it's worth the effort, of course, but if a man practices he might find he can eventually do it easily, allowing him to climax and then have dry orgasms afterwards." The method I'm about to describe works the usual way, by learning how to *prevent* ejaculation. "We are convinced," write Hartman and Fithian, "that the only obstacles to a man's experiencing multiple orgasms of one kind or another are his conditioning and his acceptance of the idea that for a man orgasm and ejaculation always come together."

Finally, before getting on to the program, how long will it take? The answer is—it depends. It depends on how strong your PC muscle is. It depends on how determined you are to succeed. It depends on how calm you are during sex, and the sort of relationship you have with your partner—it will work faster if you have a close, supportive relationship in which the sex is relaxed and mutually enjoyable. Hartman had one man who taught himself to become multiorgasmic in a single week. For most it will take between two and eight weeks.

STEP ONE:

Strengthening Your PC Muscle

The first thing to do is locate your PC muscle, which runs between the pubic bone at the front and the coccyx, or tailbone, at the back. The simplest way to do this is to try to stop the flow of urine next time you go to the bathroom. The muscle you have to tense for this is the PC muscle, and it is best to try to control the flow of urine with it while you're sitting down, so that you can learn how to do the exercises when sitting anywhere. It is also the muscle a man uses to make his penis wiggle around when he's playing the goat. Hartman and Fithian cite an obnoxious-sounding schoolboy who grew so strong that he "could hang a towel on his penis before and after gym, much to the amusement of his friends, and he would make the towel move by tensing his PC muscle."

Kegel exercises consist simply of getting this PC muscle into shape, in the same way one would tone up any other muscle, by repeatedly contracting and relaxing it. At first, before you've gotten adept at the exercises, you may find yourself tensing your buttocks and stomach at the same time as your PC. Don't. This is not a bottom or beer-belly exercise. Try doing the Kegels while sitting on a hard chair. If there's any indication that you're up to something peculiar—e.g., if you're rising up and down on the seat or going purple in the face from lack of air—you've got the wrong part of the body. When properly done, Kegel exercises can be performed in the middle of a crowded room, on the bus, in an elevator, or while giving a lecture to the Women's Institute, without anybody knowing a thing about it.

There are two types of exercises, and both are important.

Kegel Exercise One: Contract and release the PC muscle rapidly. The plan requires that you slowly build up the number of these you do every day, until you can eventually manage 200 a day. These should not be done all at once, but in groups of ten or twenty.

Kegel Exercise Two: Contract the PC muscle and hold for three seconds, then release for three seconds. Again, eventually you want to do 200 of these a day, in groups. In both cases, the chart at the end of the chapter explains how to build up to this number over a two-week period.

Like any other muscle in the body, keeping the PC well toned is good for your health. Even if you don't want to become multiorgasmic, you should contract and relax this muscle at least fifty times every day. Let it go flabby, and you will have not only much less control over your ejaculation, but also poor bladder and bowel control. A well-exercised PC protects against prostate disease and impotence. Congested arteries in the pelvic area reduce blood flow, which makes it harder for a man to get and maintain an erection. Kegel exercises force more blood through the capillaries, which cleans away the gunge, increasing circulation. Some men claim that Kegels have also increased their penis size.

The main trouble with Kegels is remembering to do them. They are such slight, dull little things that it's quite possible, despite best intentions, to forget all about them for days at a time. Get into the habit of doing them at certain times of day, such as before and after meals, during the commercials on TV, in the bath, on the way to work, between pints of Guinness at the pub. After two or three days, you'll automatically associate the exercises with these activities, and will no longer forget to do your quota. Tom:

> As a real estate agent I'm on the phone a lot talking to clients, and now the ringing immediately makes me think that I should be moving my member at the same time, at the same pace. I keep them up sometimes dur-

ing the whole time I'm working out Mrs. A's mortgage or Mr. B's bridging loan. I call them my pelvic clients. I'm Charles Atlas of the groin!

If you feel very sore the day after doing a set of Kegel exercises, don't push yourself. You can do more damage than good by suddenly overstraining a muscle that is in a lazy, weak condition. You must work gradually. Reduce the number of exercises, and start to increase them again only when the soreness disappears. By the end of the program, you'll be doing (with ease) about 200 repetitions of each exercise every day.

STEP TWO:

Learning to Have Multiple Orgasms on Your Own

As well as doing the Kegels every day to build up muscular control of ejaculation, you must train your body using masturbation. The approach follows on from the masturbation exercises in Step Two of the last chapter, in which you learned how to delay your climax for as long as your lover wants. Now, the idea is to bring yourself as near to climax as possible, without actually going over. As your control and self-awareness develop, you will be able to get closer and closer to the critical moment and then use your PC muscle to prevent ejaculation. Eventually you will be adept enough to have an orgasm while still withholding your semen. This is all you have to learn.

Note: For men who have difficulty lasting more than fifteen or twenty minutes during intercourse, go back to chapter 12 and work through those exercises until you have learned basic control. The exercises in this chapter represent the advanced level. Without having mastered the basics, it is as precipitate to plunge ahead with them as it would be to take trigonometry without knowing algebra.

The Exercises

As before, find yourself a nice, quiet place where you're not going to be disturbed.

1. Masturbate until you feel very close to climax (but not so close as to make it inevitable) and then tense your PC muscle to bring your ejaculation under control. Don't go at this in a fast and furious fashion, rubbing your member until it glows: do it gently. The point is to develop government of your responses, not create a nasty mess in record time.

Do this exercise several times in a session, each time trying to get a little closer to the point at which orgasm becomes inevitable, and then shying away just short of it by stopping the stimulation and contracting your PC muscle. The timing is difficult, and the temptation to get on and get satisfied is great. But control yourself. Learning not to give in to the easy temptation is part of the exercise. If you do misjudge the timing, don't worry. Simply try to be more precise the next time you find yourself on your own.

Do this exercise two or three times during the first week, getting close and backing off five times each (and, after that, do as you like), until you feel fully in command of your climax— i.e., no more mistakes or very near mistakes. During the second week, progress to . . .

2. As Exercise 1, but this time end up by masturbating gently beyond the point when orgasm becomes inevitable, and then try to prevent ejaculation by tensing your PC muscle. At first, you're unlikely to succeed. This is not only because it takes time to develop strength and control, but also because it takes time to work out what sort of control works for you. Some men say that repeated contraction of their PC is the most effective means of preventing ejaculation; others insist, on the contrary, that this promotes ejaculation more than ever, and that the only way is to keep the muscle constantly tense during climax.

There are two other methods of preventing ejaculation

that you can also use. They are awkward and suitable only for masturbation, but until you figure out how to work with your PC alone, they are extremely useful. The first is the squeeze technique. It was invented by Masters and Johnson as a technique for curing premature ejaculation, in which the woman squeezed her partner's member every time he felt ejaculation getting close. It is illustrated in the edition I have of their book by two feminine fingers with sharp nails—the penis looks, poor thing, like a fish about to have its gills gouged out. It can be just as easily done by the owner of the penis. The idea is to block the tube up which the semen travels, by squeezing firmly, just below the head of the penis, between two fingers and a thumb.

The second method of preventing ejaculation is to prevent your testicles from rising. It is a little-known trick, and a very nifty one. When a man gets aroused, the scrotal sac tightens, lifting the testicles against his body. He can't ejaculate unless they're in that position. So, to prevent ejaculation, all he has to do is prevent them from getting there by whatever manner takes his fancy. Some men hold their testicles between their legs, though this requires a certain looseness. Others grab (gently!) and hold down. A third approach is to push your fingers against the scrotal sac between penis and testicles, and push them away. Nigel:

This worked the first time for me. Mary had gone out and I was feeling frustrated so I started . . . you know. When I was about to come, I pushed my hand down to hold my balls away and tensed my love muscles. I came, but there was hardly any semen at all. I could have been satisfied with that but then, for the first time ever, I knew I didn't have to be. My penis got a bit less hard afterwards, but I kept going—more out of curiosity than anything else, really—and about five minutes later came again.

Practice with all these approaches to see which works best for you. As Nigel mentioned, you may find that your penis loses a bit of firmness after climaxing the first time, and that there may be some semen—don't worry on either count. What matters is that you feel you can go on. Study your breathing as well. Some men find that by holding their breath, or breathing very rapidly as they get close to climaxing, they have greater control over their ejaculation.

Once you've finished this exercise, you will have had several multiple orgasms, and it will be time to move on to having them with your partner. This may take anything from a week to a couple of months, depending on how well developed your PC is, and how loyal you are to the exercise plan. Don't worry if you fail many times: the body has to be reconditioned and this takes time. Eventually you will succeed.

STEP THREE:

Learning to Have Multiple Orgasms with Your Partner

If you have perfected Step Two, and can now separate ejaculation from orgasm using your PC muscle alone, then transferring your ability to intercourse will be comparatively easy. There are more things going on to distract you when you're having sex with another person, and it may take a while to get as much control over your responses as you have during masturbation, but with practice you will soon get the knack. There are no exercises to perform in this step, but there are a few points to bear in mind.

1. Position. A consideration only at first, while you're still getting the hang of how to use your PC muscles. The best position depends on how much stiffness your penis momentarily loses after each climax. If it's a great deal, then it's better that you should be on top, or else the little fellow will drop out. Otherwise, it's better with your partner on top. This makes it easier for you to relax and concentrate on controlling yourself, and for her to provide exactly the sort of stimulation you both need.

2. Contracting her PC muscle. Women have a PC muscle just like men (see chapter 7 for further discussion of this), which is useful both for improving the quality of their orgasms and for creating greater friction during intercourse. It is also good for holding on to a penis that has just climaxed and making sure it stays erect and can't escape. Get her to tense her PC as you tense yours, so that she can continue to give the penis maximum, gentle stimulation during the moments after your orgasm.

3. Remember, multiple orgasms are NOT the best thing sex has to offer. The man who can climax five times without ever stopping intercourse is a pain in the neck if he doesn't excite his partner at the same time. A man who can climax only once will be a far better companion if he can control the moment at which he comes and makes the sex stimulating for her.

On the next page you'll see a chart to guide you through the first two weeks. I suggest beginning this minute with fifty repetitions of each of the Kegel exercises, and make tomorrow day two. Don't do more than fifty, and concentrate on doing them properly. Altogether, it will take up six minutes of your time. So, put down the book now, get the exercises over with, then read on . . .

THE CHART FOR MULTIPLE ORGASM EXERCISES

	Step One		Step Two	Step Three
Day	Kegel 1	Kegel 2	On Your Own	With Your Partner (Note the results)
1	50	50		
2	50	50	Exercise One	
3	75	75		
4	75	75	Exercise One	
5	100	100		
6	100	100	Exercise One	
7	125	125		
8	125	125		
9	150	150	Exercise Two	
10	150	150		
11	175	175	Exercise Two	
12	175	175		
13	200	200	Exercise Two	
14	200	200		

NOTE: This chart represents a guide only. It should be modified to suit your circumstances and fitness. It is unlikely that you will learn to become fully multiorgasmic within two weeks, so do not despair just because you've gotten to the last line in the chart without success. Continue doing 200 repetitions of each of the Kegel exercises per day, and concentrate on improving your control during masturbation, until you do succeed.

14

Danger!

*S*exual harassment and date rape have become big subjects in the last decade. Heavy new analyses regularly appear in the gender studies section of the bookstore. Every week we read in the newspaper about women (and, occasionally, men) who've lost their jobs or are suing their bosses because of some form of sexual misconduct. Universities in America are actually suggesting that couples sign a contract before going out on a date, explaining what each expects from the other! Outraged polemicists are everywhere. Men don't know what the hell is going on.

Yet the majority of men are perfectly able to judge what is reasonable and what is not. For those of you wanting a little more clarity about the issue I offer here a few guidelines.

Sexual Harassment

Sexual harassment comes in many forms, from suggestive comments and wolf whistles to physical assault. At best it is a minor irritation, part of the rough and tumble of daily life, and at the extreme end it is rape. Most of the time it is degrading to both parties.

Women are much more sensitive to unwanted sexual intimacies than men, because men are stronger than women and their sex drive is more brutal. Men often don't appreciate just how unpleasant leering, suggestive conversation, and unwanted contact can be because they think of it in terms of how they'd like to be approached by a forward woman. But this gives a completely false picture of the way women actually feel. Such behavior is as unpleasant to a woman as it would be for a heterosexual man in a locker room full, not of seductresses, but of homosexual weight lifters. A woman has only her wit, which usually has to be used against superior numbers, to get herself out of a difficult situation. A man can, and not infrequently does, back up his innuendo with physical force. Says Louisa:

> Aggressive sexual attention from more than one man is particularly unpleasant—passing a construction site, or in an all-male office. They are making clear their desire to fuck me, and there is no doubt that they *could* if they chose, against my will. Of course in most situations you know it won't happen, but that's not the point. It *could* and it's as if they were reminding you of that. You can feel very vulnerable.

I read recently of one man, quite a big tough fellow, who found himself the only male in a factory full of women. They made his life such hell with sexual harassment that he had a nervous breakdown.

Much sexual harassment is not physical at all, but involves a man being verbally intrusive. Some of it is not even intentional, no more than flirtatious pleasantry in the hands of a social Ostrogoth. I witnessed a typical example in a college bar recently. A man—we'll call him Robert—was sitting at a table drinking with some friends. He was popular with most people, chatty, and, though married, known to be a "woman's man." He ogled women persistently and sex was never far from his conversation, in a friendly sort of way. Quite late in the evening an attractive, twenty-six-year-old female graduate student came in.

"Hello, Rosalind," said Robert. "You look different today."

"I've had my hair cut."

"Mm," responded Robert quickly. "Wish you'd give me a cut and blow job."

He thought this wildly humorous. So did two of his male friends. The others, and all the women, found it disgusting. It wasn't funny, it was intrusive and it made Rosalind feel she couldn't talk with Robert, whom she quite liked, because everyone was thinking about her sucking him off. The idea revolted her. She had to leave. Robert couldn't understand it.

Miss J. M., from London, described another situation. It is much more severe but, again, familiar to many women. J. M. is intelligent, efficient, attractive, has a steady boyfriend, and works in a small, male-dominated office. Yet from the first day of the job a selection of the men who worked with her started making comments about the size of her breasts. "The first remark was so unexpected it was in a way the worst. Here I was, a full-grown woman in an important job with responsibilities, a house, a taxpayer, a car of my own, a degree in natural sciences. And a middle-aged man says: 'You've got big *assets*. You should share them with me.' I felt like I had come out of the city and into a zoo . . ."

Over the next few weeks it got worse and worse. It wasn't just the cumulative effect, but they were sort of winding themselves up. If they got away with one thing, then next time they'd try something a little bit more daring. A *Playboy* spread in my drawer one week would, unless I protested, be upgraded to an accidentally-on-purpose touch the next. My boyfriend wanted to kill them. Finally, after lots of heart-searching, I complained.

At which point a lot of sexually harassed women lose their jobs, while the men who made their lives so unpleasant get a tiny reprimand. It happens every day of the week. But J. M. was lucky:

> I was pretty certain that I'd lose my job as a result. Instead, the boss was really great. He brought the men in and tore them apart. He really understood the problem. One of them had been complained about lots of times before, so he fired him. He couldn't afford to have this contempt in his office. Of course they didn't admit it. They squirmed away from the issue and said, "But it was only flattery, you shouldn't be so uptight," or "We were just treating her like one of the boys." One of the boys! No man ever went up to the men and said show us your dick so I can suck it, but I'm supposed to be flattered when a slob suggests he wants to put his face in my cleavage. I wanted to be sick. It was like they had two languages. One for me when I was at my desk, and the other for themselves and the outside world, whenever they were called on to explain their behavior. The wife of the fired one was sent a letter explaining the reasons for his dismissal. She divorced him not long afterwards.

The sexual harasser is less than a man. What he does demeans him. Women are much less confrontational than men and often suffer such treatment in silence rather than risk "nastiness" by complaining. But they notice, and they talk about it with their friends (male and female). The man whose conversation revolves around sex and making intimate remarks to every nubile woman he sets his eyes on (there's one of them who lives near me) will soon make himself ridiculous to everyone in town.

A milder example is a male friend of mine who makes a

habit, when talking to a woman, of taking her by the hand. It is a very small presumption on his part, but I wish he wouldn't do it. It is sexually motivated and I don't like the enforced intimacy. Once again, when trying to judge whether something you do might be regarded as unpleasant, imagine a known homosexual man doing it to you. (Incidentally, this example is *in no sense* intended as anti-homosexual: it is the only way to make a reasonable approximation to what women feel.) If it would make you uncomfortable, then you're straying into risky territory. Whether the woman you are speaking to will also regard it as disagreeable depends on how close and easy your relationship with her is. Women, like men, vary greatly in what they find acceptable.

Here are a few more points to bear in mind.

1. Avoid all intimate sexual comments or insinuations. "You look gorgeous" is presumptuous, but probably okay in informal situations. "Your breasts are particularly pert today" is never acceptable. Looks and gestures are equally unpleasant, if not more so, because the woman has nothing solid to reply to. When more than one man is involved it is particularly distressing. A man *knows* when he has intended a remark or gesture to be sexual, so if challenged or if she seems distressed don't be a rat and deny it, or ignore it: have the courage to come clean and apologize. I would think a great deal of a man who, after realizing he had gone too far, followed it with, "I'm sorry, that was out of order. I apologize."

2. Beware of repeated comments or gestures. Many things are okay once, but become tiresome or threatening when kept up. And, as above, be particularly vigilant when there is more than one man likely to offend. Knowing two people are snickering about you together is utterly unpleasant. Or the problem may be one of men acting not together, but cumulatively. Heather:

Last week in the office a man I know was passing and
made a small suggestive comment. He was totally
shocked when I snapped and let fly at him . . . To him
it seemed a mild thing, but actually I had already had
three such approaches that day. If you stop and think
about it, you realize that even a tenth of what women
are expected to endure would seriously anger a man.

3. Most of all, be alert to her responses. Not the least humiliating aspect of sexual harassment for women is when somebody
willfully ignores one's distress. Some women enjoy playful comments back and forth, but when she responds with silence it
does *not* mean she approves. Don't push the point. Nor is it
enough to excuse any remark as "only a joke." Many a deeply
upset woman has also been accused of being a "killjoy" or having "no sense of humor." A joke is not automatically a joke because it is intended as such. If it gives offense, it is merely an
unpleasant remark and therefore always demands an apology,
not further insult.

Date Rape

The simple definition of date rape is making a woman have sex
against her will, during a date. In most cases—i.e., those involving force or threat of force—it's different from ordinary rape
only by virtue of the circumstances. Ordinary rape comes out of
the blue. Date rape occurs in what is already a potentially sexual setting. But the case against the man is just as clear-cut. The
woman said "No," and the man went ahead and did it to her
anyway. He knows perfectly well what he's guilty of.

The difficulties crop up when the woman didn't say "No,"
or didn't say it very firmly, or said, "No" but then sort of hinted
that "No" might mean "Yes." She may call it rape, but the man
might honestly insist that the sex was consensual in the end,

even if she showed a little reluctance at first. Once again, no one could possibly set down a definitive code of conduct on these points. All I can hope to do is give a few guidelines.

Imagine, for example, that you've just met an attractive woman and gotten an invitation up to her apartment. You managed to speak up just in time and suggest a cup of coffee. In the living room you arrange matters so that you sit side by side on the sofa. What next?

You search secretly for signs of interest and aren't sure. So you pursue the intimacy by increments, and eventually find you have gotten ahold of her hand. If this far enough? Should you venture a kiss, or return to your own apartment for an ice-cold bath and a determined read of the *Critique of Pure Reason*? Once kissed, she might yield other favors. You try it. She protests. You keep trying; she keeps protesting; but eventually you get your way. In order to encourage her a bit, you point out that a kiss is only a kiss. It's just a show of fondness—nothing major. You try it again, with some persistence, and again you get your way. You congratulate yourself for having thrown on an extra dollop of aftershave and given your bottle of Manly ("perfume of intimacy") a shake in the appropriate places. You touch her neck. She ducks away a little, but doesn't actually slap your face or push you off. You touch her breast. Again she protests, but gives in when you remark that she shouldn't feel prudish about her assets. You go the whole hog, and she lies there, receptive till the final gasp.

It is only when you're padding around the apartment looking for tissues that she stands up and spits in your face. "I feel sick, soiled, disgusting!" she screams. "You've just raped me! How can you walk around as if that were nothing?" Ten minutes later she calls the police.

The conclusion is difficult here. You did not use force to get your way, and when the woman points out in court that she did say "No," you can retort that it was hardly a firm "No." After all, during foreplay with a new partner there is always a bit of play and testing. How were you to learn what her weak "No" really meant unless you pushed the matter a bit further? This is a plausible argument. Maybe her negative was just coquetry or the last breath of some needless scruple.

Nevertheless, you have committed rape.

Today women are more sexually liberated than ever before and quite capable of encouraging sex when they really do want it. Therefore anyone who does not give an explicit "Yes" to sex, whether verbal or physical, *must* be assumed to be discouraging it. A man runs the risk of getting himself into very deep trouble if he pretends otherwise. The woman's passivity, in our case, was a sign of her despair, not her approval. Male persistence is extraordinarily wearing and difficult to withstand, particularly if you like the man. How many times was it necessary for her to say "No"? Once should have been enough, but a dozen times were not. You raped her because you were so carried away you refused to pay attention to the signs. You placed her in an unpleasant all-or-nothing situation: she must go all the way or make a big scene and ruin the evening. Many, many women will recognize that, in the mood of the moment, it is simpler to give in. I know many women who have ended up having sex against their will because of the sheer persistence and emotional pressure of the man.

Here is a real example taken from Shere Hite of the situation from the woman's point of view:

> One guy I felt really excited about. I made a date with him, thinking we would get together to drink and talk, walk around a little. It turned out he assumed I would come up to his place. I still wanted to give him the benefit of the doubt, not thinking he could possibly try to push anything *that* fast. I was disappointed in his apartment when one move led to another—just like all the other guys—sitting me on the couch, giving me a drink, taking off my shoes, giving me a pillow, lying next to me,

holding my hand, then pressing himself to me. I could have gotten up at any stage, but it is just like paralysis, they always accuse you of making a scene over "nothing" if you get up after one of these little stages, and then if you get up after one of the big stages, they claim you are a cockteaser, why did you go so far? And now just to leave them there like this . . . ? Anyway, I got into that old college thing and just lay there not believing the pumping away that he did. I just wished it were over so I could get away, but I was unable to tell him.

Sex by increments is very popular with some men. The woman begins as a "prude" if she will not yield to small attentions, and ends as a "cocktease" if she pulls back from full sex. Young women are especially vulnerable to this unpleasant tactic. When Hite's subject says, "I just wished it were over so I could get away, but I was unable to tell him," it may sound feeble to an outsider, but it masks a dead weight of unpleasant feelings engendered by that evening.

Here is an example of something that brought home to me just how vulnerable women—especially sexually inexperienced women—can be. When I was sixteen, I got a job at a theatrical club in London, serving drinks and dinner. One evening an actor came in. He was about twenty-eight, good-looking, and all the rest. We got into a long discussion about life and art and poetry. He was an intense character, and at one point started insisting that everything in life is either black or white. There are no in-betweens, he said. "Wow! profound!" I thought, and agreed enthusiastically. Later, fondling in his apartment, I made it clear that I didn't want to sleep with him. He was furious. All that black and white nonsense of his had actually been about sex: a sixteen-year-old schoolgirl should be prepared either to fuck a man or not touch him at all. When the taxi came, he remarked: "You're lucky I'm not insisting. Most men wouldn't give you any choice." I was supposed to congratulate him that he hadn't raped me.

Forcing a woman to have sex doesn't necessarily mean the use of physical force. A man might, for example, blackmail a woman into going to bed with him. He might say, "Unless you fuck me, I'll get you fired from work." That's a surprisingly popular tactic with rapists. As I write, the newspapers are full of the case of an Olympic swimming coach who systematically raped young swimmers over years and years—he ensured their silence by fear, and by the fact that he held great power over their life's ambitions. The rapist might be less extreme about it and say that "Unless you fuck me, I'll spread disgusting rumors about you." Or he may not make his threat explicit, but allow it to be understood that unless the woman complies with what he wants—which is, after all, just a brief five minutes of (hopefully) painless activity—he will give her months and months of emotional punishment.

A man can never be completely sure that he will not be *called* a rapist, as unfortunately a few women change their minds *after* the event. But he can be completely sure that he never *is* a rapist by observing a single rule:

"NO" ALWAYS MEANS "NO."

There lingers a long-held belief that women say "No" when they really mean "Yes." It stems from two misconceptions: the idea that females are muddle-headed, silly, and not capable of being practical; and the notion that it is becoming to their maidenly modesty to be reticent in sex.

A delightful example of this ridiculous misconception appears in Jane Austen's masterpiece *Pride and Prejudice,* published in 1813. The repulsive sycophantic clergyman Mr. Collins proposes marriage to the lovely and very firm-minded heroine Elizabeth Bennet, who promptly douses cold water on the idea. Mr. Collins, far from being deflated, is actively encouraged:

"I am not now to learn," replied Mr Collins, with a formal wave of the hand, "that it is usual with young ladies to reject the addresses of the man whom they secretly mean to accept, when he first applies for their favour; and that sometimes the refusal is repeated a second or even a third time. I am therefore by no means discouraged by what you have just said, and shall hope to lead you to the altar ere long."

Again, Elizabeth insists that she knows her own mind and her "No" means "No." "You must give me leave to judge for myself, and pay me the compliment of believing what I say." Mr. Collins is unfazed. "When I do myself the honour of speaking to you next on this subject I shall hope to receive a more favourable answer than you have now given me; though I am far from accusing you of cruelty at present . . . perhaps you have even now said as much to encourage my suit as would be consistent with the true delicacy of the female character."

Elizabeth warmly repeats that she does not want the odious man, at any price. "You are uniformly charming!" exclaims Mr. Collins, "and I am persuaded that when sanctioned by the express authority of both your excellent parents, my proposals will not fail of being acceptable."

Behind all the no-means-yes scenarios lies a hopeful interpretation of what the woman really wants. By his greater wisdom the insistent man exposes her true needs. That repellent phrase, "I made a woman out of her" means that "if it hadn't been for my overcoming the physical (and emotional) barriers of her virginity/reluctance, she'd still be cocooned in some halfformed state." It is the stuff of pornography. Ordinary females are perfectly capable of saying what they mean. When a woman opens her lips into a sort of oval, tongue pressed against upper teeth, and says firmly "No," that means stop. She doesn't want you to go on. If she says it weakly or falteringly, then you should confirm that she's not playing the coquette by asking her outright, "Do you really want me to stop?" If she says "Yes" then you must stop.

Which brings us, once more, back to you and the woman who has just accused you of rape.

Unless you get that explicit consent for sex with a woman you've just taken out on a date, you must not be surprised if she hauls you up for it afterward. She didn't want sex and gave you no active encouragement; yet you had it with her. You may have been innocent of any evil intention, or you may have been a skunk, but unless you follow this rule of conduct, you're playing with fire. It might even be that she's the guilty one. Women often get drunk and go to bed with men they wouldn't usually touch with a ten-foot pole; and a rare few of them—disgraces to our sex—will afterward try to convince themselves that they weren't to blame by accusing the man of date rape. There's nothing you can do about this except be cautious always, and doubly cautious when the woman's too drunk to get her clothes off without your help.

There is only one situation in which both protagonists can safely be assumed to mean the opposite of what they say . . .

Woman (*her cheeks flushed and undoing her blouse*): No, we mustn't.

Man (*pulling off his shoes, undoing his belt*): No, no, think of my children.

Woman (*releasing her breasts, pulling back the bed-sheets*): No, really. I love my husband.

Man (*moistening his organ*): No, no, no!

15

Rolling Off

*J*ust as women become sexually aroused gradually, so they also cool down gradually. Even after she has climaxed a dozen times and is perfectly satisfied, a woman still takes a while to come down from her high. It is therefore an unpleasant shock if the man reacts to his own orgasm as he would to a brick wall, coming to an abrupt halt and collapsing into frigid sleep.

For many women, the period just after orgasm is the most important moment. It is the time of greatest emotional intimacy, when the gentle, companionable side of sex takes center stage, uncomplicated by the physical urge for penetration and climax. Whether you're a new partner who hopes to be remembered and invited back, a gigolo who wants to further his reputation, or a husband who wishes to spice up his marriage, afterward is one of the best times to advance the cause.

How you actually go about behaving after sex is over is, of course, your own business, but there are certain rules of etiquette. Strangely, very few sex books even mention this vastly important subject. Women are constantly lamenting how often their partners overlook it.

Postcoital Etiquette

Like all good manners, the purpose of postcoital etiquette is to make the other person feel both comfortable and valued. The man's first consideration, therefore, is to:

1. Find out if She Is Satisfied. But don't do it by asking the dreaded "Didjacum?" question. It's blunt and smacks of oneupmanship. Much as you are longing to know the answer, it is to intercourse what the question "What's a nice girl like you doing in a business like this?" is to prostitution: the oldest, most hackneyed thing in the book. A better method is to say, in a gentle voice as you extract yourself and return to lying beside your beloved, "Is there something more I could do for you?" or "Would you like me to keep on a little?" This volunteering approach can be dressed up in all sorts of guises, such as: "Please, please feel free to take advantage of your sex slave for as long as you want."

If she answers, without significant hesitation, "No," then all is well and good. If she hesitates, press the point until you get a response you can trust.

An unequivocal "Yes" means you have to fulfill your duties. Even if you are dying to go to sleep and feel as far away from sexual desire as from the moon, you *must* rouse yourself if you want to gain good lover status. Even premature ejaculation can be overlooked if you are prepared to satisfy her some other way. In fact, many women prefer nonpenetrative satisfaction. Bernadette:

> In itself there's nothing wrong with a man who comes quickly as long as he doesn't think that sex ends for me at the same time. As long as he does something about it. I don't particularly like being penetrated anyway so I'm happy when my husband stops using his penis and

goes back to doing something else to satisfy me after he's orgasmed.

Manual sex is the easiest and the most attractive option, but *please* be sure to make it quite clear that you enjoy doing it and find it exciting to watch her getting aroused. It's not enough that you *do* enjoy it, you must *show* that you enjoy it.

Postcoital oral sex has an obvious drawback if you didn't use a condom, though some men don't mind. The third approach is not to withdraw at all, but to lie still and let her stimulate her clitoris by moving her hips beneath you. Jackie:

> I do this sometimes with James and it works very well. I find it sexy because his dick is going limp and soft and he is lying on top of me like a baby, very weak, so I can rotate my pelvis slowly. Even if his penis drops out it doesn't matter because it's really just like manual sex but using the man's whole body instead of his hand.

This technique works well only in the missionary position. When it is clear that you are both fully satisfied (or, at least, that you've both had enough) the following points of etiquette become important:

2. Mopping Up. The famous wet patch. Since the most popular sexual position is the missionary, in which the man lies on top of the woman on the woman's side of the bed, it is she who always ends up sleeping with an area of cold, gooey fluid sticky against her thigh. Decency demands that you take an interest in this patch, e.g., find some tissues or a towel to lay over the offending region. The gallant lover will take care that sex occurs on his side of the bed at least half of the time.

3. Smoking. The postcoital cigarette is all very well if both of you are smokers, but quite disgusting if one of you is not. Cigarette smoke impregnates your breath, her hair, the bedclothes, the whole room, and it stays there with the tenacity of a leech. *Always* have the courtesy to ask if she minds, before lighting up. If it's her bed you are sleeping in, try hard to desist altogether, and if you can't, smoke out of the window.

The reason women often get angry when men light up after sex is not simply the smell, but the fact that smoking is a cold gesture. A person with a cigarette seems to put most of his concentration on that long white tube, and have little left over for the woman he's just made love to.

4. Going to Sleep. Don't do it right away. You don't have to lie awake for hours, but you should show that your partner still means something to you now that the vigorous part is over. THIS IS VERY IMPORTANT. Keep touching her, hold her hand, stroke her hair, her body. Julie:

> . . . afterwards we lie in each other's arms. This is the happiest time for me. I like for him to be in contact and to feel his body warm against mine while his penis gets small and sweet again. He strokes my back and plays with my hair so that I get lulled into a sleep which is very very relaxed. When I wake up the next morning I remember how good the sex was with him and am furious that I have to go back home. From the moment I meet him until the moment I wake up the next day, I feel as though it has all been lovemaking. He makes me melt because he fulfills all I want from a passionate lover so much.
>
> I wouldn't say John is a bad lover but he is not an intimate lover. I don't think I'm getting something from John that I could not get from somebody else. An intimate lover makes a lot of contact with his woman whereas John only does what's strictly necessary and afterwards he doesn't do anything at all. I want him to be

more than his penis but I can't make him understand this. I just want a cuddle.

When you do at last fall asleep, make sure it seems as if it's something you want to do *with* her, not separately: a bit of uncomfortable snoozing face-to-face, before turning over to find your most comfortable position.

5. Doing Things Together. Instead of sleeping immediately, it's far sexier and more intimate (especially for new couples) to stay awake and do something together. Karen:

> When I first met Alec we made love three times in a row, and it was still only midnight. I was feeling drowsy and very pleasant. Alec got up and told me to keep dozing. I thought he'd gone to have a bath, but half an hour later he burst in with a tray . . . he'd been through my fridge and concocted a meal with all the odd ingredients he could find! I remember how we sat up in bed, wrapped in the blanket, with Nina Simone playing, eating some peculiar fish tacos with oodles of melted cheese. It was the most romantic, pleasurable evening I have ever had. It was such a nice, such an unexpected thing for him to do.

Nina spent an evening of passion with Freddie and, when they found that neither was sleepy . . .

> We sat up and played a game a bit like ludo. It's a traditional Indian board game. But the wonderful part is, the board was a design sewn into an Indian bedcover that Freddie had. He'd bought it in India. Now that's cool. I shall remember Freddie and the board game for a long time.

Sarah, on the other hand, had had a pleasant time in bed with Martin but was totally turned off him because . . .

> As soon as we'd finished he put on his robe and went over to the telephone. It was about nine o'clock and we were in his apartment. He started making telephone calls, lots of them. His mind was already miles away, planning what he was going to do tomorrow. He didn't even say "Excuse me, but this is a really urgent call" (which they evidently weren't). I can't tell you how cold that made me feel. I hated him.

Tracey had a completely different experience:

> After we'd made love Rickie told me to get dressed in some old jeans of his and a dirty sweater. It was way past midnight and he took a flashlight and led me out-side, down to the bottom of his garden. I was wonder-ing what sort of pervert's den he had down there, I was expecting porno videos or something. He opened the door and shone the flashlight in, and there were a hun-dred pairs of little red eyes looking at me. They were his pigeons, he was a pigeon-lover. The way he loved those birds made me look at him with new eyes. It may not sound like a sexy scenario, but it was magic be-cause he was sharing this magical rapport with me. I know no other man will show me that.

6. The Next Day. This applies particularly to flings and first-time lovers. Even if you intend not to see each other again, it is still important to make a gesture the next day. Women spend a large part of their time trying to avoid men who "want them only for the sex," so show that the whole thing meant some-thing to you by phoning or sending a letter.

If you send flowers, take care over the message. Write

something personal—the message is much more important than the flowers, which, though nice, are pretty standard morning-after fare. I fully agree with Josie's view:

> I know some women are thrilled by red roses, but I personally find them corny. Because they are a standard "romantic" gesture, he hasn't had to think. I'd rather have something unusual that is special to me. Nice gestures don't have to be expensive, they only have to show you've given it some thought.

The point about morning-after gestures is to say that what went on the evening before was special. One man I knew sent his paramour a bowl of pineapples along with a lengthy love letter after their first night together. Another, now in the twelfth year of his marriage, swears that the reason he and his wife are so happy together is because they always have a "bit of cuddle and closeness the morning after" before getting up. There's nothing erotic about it, "But it shows that we're together and that it means something. Not that we think about it consciously like that, it just happens that way, because it makes the day nice to follow. Quite honestly, I don't think I could get to work without it sometimes!"

And now, Good Luck! I hope you have great success in the future—and don't forget to send me your completed questionnaire (via the publisher).

About the Author

DIDO DAVIES grew up in Chelsea, London, in the swinging sixties, at a time when attitudes toward sex were changing dramatically. She gained her Ph.D. in English literature at the University of Cambridge, where, at Emmanuel College, she was one of the first women students since it was founded in 1584. Her biography of the comic novelist William Gerhardie won a national literary prize. As well as sex, she writes about history and is currently completing a classic English murder mystery.

ALEXANDER MASTERS was born in Manhattan and has worked as an independent sex researcher for nine years. He is also a travel writer, science book reviewer, mathematics teacher, and fundraiser for the homeless. He has appeared as a sex expert on the English television show *The Good Sex Guide*.

How to Have an Orgasm . . . As Often As You Want was an international bestseller, translated into seventeen languages. Alexander and Dido chose the pseudonym RACHEL SWIFT in order to distinguish the sex guides from their other writing. And also, in view of the explicit nature of the Rachel Swift books, to spare the blushes of their families.